Quality at home for older people

Involving service users in defining home care specifications

Norma Raynes, Bogusia Temple, Charlotte Glenister and Lydia Coulthard

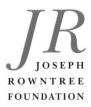

JOSEPH
ROWNTREE
FOUNDATION

First published in Great Britain in June 2001 by

The Policy Press
34 Tyndall's Park Road
Bristol BS8 1PY
UK

Tel no +44 (0)117 954 6800
Fax no +44 (0)117 973 7308
E-mail tpp@bristol.ac.uk
www.policypress.org.uk

Published for the Joseph Rowntree Foundation by The Policy Press

ISBN 1 86134 352 3

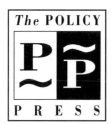

Norma Raynes is Professor of Social Care, **Bogusia Temple** is Senior Research Fellow, **Charlotte Glenister** and **Lydia Coulthard** are Research Assistants, all in the Institute for Health and Social Care Research in the Faculty of Health and Social Care, University of Salford.

The **Joseph Rowntree Foundation** has supported this project as part of its programme of research and innovative development projects, which it hopes will be of value to policy makers, practitioners and service users. The facts presented and views expressed in this report are, however, those of the authors and not necessarily those of the Foundation.

Designed by Adkins Design, York
Printed in Great Britain by Hobbs the Printers Ltd, Southampton

Contents

Acknowledgements

This research has taken place in the City of Manchester. It could not have been done without the willingness to participate in research of the City Council and the helpfulness of particular members of staff in the Department of Social Services. These colleagues, along with other local people, formed a local Steering Group. The members of this Steering Group were:

Ms Doreen Grafton, P & D Homecare Provider
Mr Ismail Lambat, Longsight/Moss Side Community Care Project
Mr Latif, Elderly Asian Development Group
Mr Kevin O'Neil, Contracts and Purchasing Unit, Manchester Social Services Department
Dr Sylvia Sham, Wai Yin Chinese Women's Society
Mr Dick Sherwood, Principal Commissioning Manager, Manchester Social Services Department
Mr Ian Thompson, Black Community Care, Afro-Caribbean Care Group
Ms Lynne White, Anchor Care Alternative

The Steering Group helped solve many of the problems that occurred during the course of the research. Equally important in enabling the research to be completed were the older people who have provided the information described in this report. Without their willingness to collaborate with the researchers, and share with us their ideas about what makes a quality home care service, this report would never have been written.

The Joseph Rowntree Foundation funded this research and we should like to thank them for that. They also provided us with an Advisory Committee who gave us necessary guidance. The members of this group were:

Charlie Barker, Social Services Director, Sefton Council
Lesley Bell, Director, Initiatives in Care
Mr Peter Dunn, Department of Health
Mr Latif, Elderly Asian Development Group
Professor Mary Marshall, Director, Dementia Services Development Centre, University of Stirling
Ms Caroline Mozley, R&D Department, York Health Services NHS Trust
Mr Alex O'Neil, Principal Research Manager, Joseph Rowntree Foundation
Mr Kevin O'Neil, Contracts and Purchasing Unit, Manchester Social Services Department

Help with the interviews and focus groups was provided by Dr B. Rawlings, Dr D. Baker and Mrs J. Gibson. Ms Christina Connolly helped with the pilot phase and literature reviews and Mrs J. Dunkerley with the early planning of the project. Mrs M. Martin helped with the organisation of the main project, and she and Mrs E. Smith helped with the typing of this manuscript.

All of these people helped us complete this difficult but immensely rewarding project.

Executive summary

Home care services provided in many local authorities include a great range of tasks. They include the provision of personal care, domestic help, aids and adaptations.

The people in our study receive home care services. They have clear views about what makes a quality home care service. The study was carried out in Manchester. Most of our findings are based on a proportionate random sample of those under and over the age of 80 receiving home care services. Some of our data derive from smaller convenience samples of people from minority groups, some but not all of whom received home care services.

Our findings describe:

1. the views and priorities about quality in home care services of those under 80 and those over 80 years of age;

2. mechanisms for accessing their views;

3. mechanisms for putting these views into practice so that they feed into the commissioning, contracting and monitoring system on a regular basis.

Older people's views on quality

When older people talk about the quality of home care services they talk about both their content and the way in which they are provided. They do not differentiate between the 'what' and the 'how' of services. Also, they do not only talk about what comes into their homes, but what enables them to get out. It is as if their view of home care is rounded, so that what happens in their home and what they experience there is affected by what they do and experience outside of it. This is not how home care providers think of home care, nor how services themselves are connected or constructed.

Older people thought that the following things were important in promoting quality in home care services:

- continuation of their existing array of personal care, domestic help, aids and adaptations to enable them to maintain their independence;

- carers doing tasks that older people identify as necessary, with a clear emphasis on more help with domestic tasks;

- provision of amenities, aids and adaptations;

- continuity of service;

- provision of information about the service;

- reliability and dependability of the service;

- monitoring the quality of the services provided;

- a responsive and sensitive quantity of provision;

- an increase in the quantity of the service when needed;

- training carers;

- improvements in the care planning process.

Older people identified additional important contributors to quality:

- the availability of safe, accessible and cheap transport;

- getting out of the house;

- improvements in health services;

- good health.

These aspects of the quality of their lives had a hugely important impact on what they felt like when they were in their homes.

There are other features of quality home care services, which were only raised by those under the age of 80. These were:

- the need for company;

- feeling safe;

- having more money.

The features of a quality home care service raised exclusively by people over the age of 80 were:

- having things to occupy your mind;

- having 'robots' to do jobs for you.

In the Chinese and Muslim communities to which we had access in Manchester, we found some overlaps with these findings. However the key finding is that information about home care services is by and large not getting to these groups. Where it is, it is because of the dedicated input of local members of these communities involved in development work. They, with support from the social services department, explain the purpose and availability of the services. There is a need to develop this kind of work and to provide information about the services in appropriate languages. Language is key in the provision of any service. It is therefore necessary to use local members of these communities directly in service provision and management. The commissioning, contracting and monitoring departments of social services need to address these issues.

Accessing older people's views and putting them into practice

Accessing ideas and putting them into practice can become a regular part of the social services' commissioning, contracting and monitoring processes. The round table discussion organised as part of this study involved older people, councillors, and senior managers from social services, health and transport agencies. At this event a number of suggestions were made to enable listening to and learning from older people to become integral to the commissioning, purchasing and monitoring of services. Those suggested here are within the power of the social services departments to action.

- Two or three times per year a patch-based round table event could be held, at which councillors, providers, senior managers and contractors come to hear people's views on current service quality. This information should then be fed into the commissioning system and the quality specifications in the contract.

- There should be a service quality specification in the care contract, which the care manager monitors by assessing one older person per provider. This may require telephone calls or visits and the use of standardised open-ended questions to record responses. The means of feeding this information into the system will need to be developed.

- The service contract should also require an annual list of the services to be made available to older people. The list should include contact details of providers, and the name and telephone number of the senior manager for adult services. For people who have reading difficulties, an audio-tape version of this information should be provided.

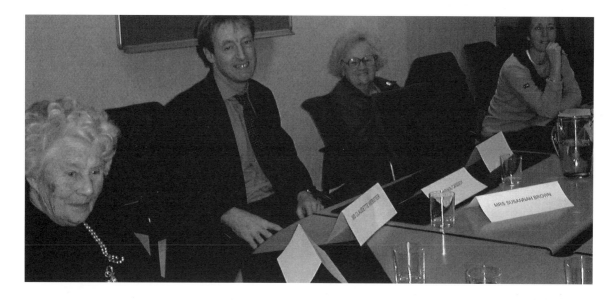

Accessing people's views about the quality of the services they receive is difficult but not impossible. It is partly affected by the accuracy of social services databases. Trying to keep these up to date is difficult for a number of reasons, not least because older people often become ill and also die.

From our findings it would appear that those who come out to meetings like the ones proposed, have similar views to those who, because of their personality, illness or disability, prefer to talk from within their own homes. There is no difference in the substantive dimensions of a quality service identified by those two groups of people. There is also overlap in how they rank the importance of the dimensions of quality home care services. However, there are differences in the priority they place on some of the identified dimensions of quality. It may therefore be worthwhile to include a small sample of people who find it difficult to get out. What is essential is the implementation of the listening and feedback process. This is a means of continuing to hear the voices of older people and act on their views of the quality of home care services.

Implications

- Some of the features of a quality service fall within the remit of the commissioning, contracting and monitoring sections of social services departments. Others do not. Those that do not are, at the local level, the responsibility of the transport department, the new Primary Care Trusts (PCTs) and the police. The views expressed by the older people in this study also have a place in the forthcoming development of national standards for the regulation and inspection of home care services (Initiatives in Care, 2000).

- The repeated identification by older people of their need for help with domestic tasks to promote quality adds to the cost of maintaining existing services. Alternative forms of this provision may need to be purchased, for example, through good neighbour schemes, or contracting with specialist cleaning companies on a block contract basis.

- The responsibility for the provision of aids or adaptations is that of both healthcare trusts and social services departments. However, the impetus for such provision often lies with social services. Primary Care Trusts and the 1999 Health Act should enable local authorities and health authorities to pool budgets or otherwise fund a service, which provides these aids and adaptations, to support people in their home (DoH, 1999). This would contribute to achieving this desirable aspect of quality in home care services. The pendants and telephones linked to call centres were highly valued by older people, but not universally known about. Basic provisions of showers, or aids to get in and out of these, and baths were also highly valued. Other adaptations such as banisters and stair-lifts are included in this category.

Twenty per cent of the people in this study appear to have no telephone. The provision of a telephone would have an impact, not only on the older person, but also on the feasibility of improvements in the organisation of services. Care managers could telephone to inform older people of changes to their service.

Other aspects of aids and adaptations raised by the older people as contributing to quality services relate to areas outside their house. These include having seats, inside and outside shops and buildings, and having doors wide enough for wheelchairs. These aspects, as with the provision of a telephone in each house, need joint working to make them feasible. It is not beyond the capability of social services departments to lead initiatives that involve telephone service providers or large supermarkets to assist in the development of public–private partnerships to achieve these ends.

What we have called the 'organisational dimensions' of home care services are areas in which social services departments can have an immediate and direct impact. They can ensure that providers inform people when changes occur. Changes will occur because of staff sickness, transport failure or other emergencies. The provision of telephones could go a long way to address this issue. Continuity of provision, that is having the same carers, is clearly of great importance to older people. Discontinuities generate anxiety for older people. If you did not know who was knocking on your door to provide personal services for you, would you open it?

The current draft of the *National standards for regulating organisations providing domiciliary care* (Initiatives in Care, 2000) addresses many of these organisational issues. This is very encouraging for older people. Setting the organisational standards is the first step towards putting in place those things that these people have identified as important contributors to a quality service. The issue for them, and for the commissioners and providers of services, is how will they all know that the new standards for these dimensions of a quality service are being implemented? We suggest some answers to this question in Chapter 6.

Transport is regarded as very important by the older people and it clearly affects the quality of their lives. It provides access to worlds outside their four walls, it enables them to continue to be and feel independent, and provides them with access to company. Older people see transport issues as relevant to the quality of home care services because access to transport affects how they feel in their own homes. These issues relating to older people's wider quality of life need to be addressed by the relevant transport authorities and the private companies providing local services. The accessibility and the flexibility of the ring-and-ride service in Manchester were greatly valued.

The longer-term vision of electronic buggies in dedicated lanes on the roads will need a strategic national approach if it is to be implemented. However, there could be pilot sites bringing health services, transport agencies and providers together, to impact on the quality of home care services for older people. The delivery of this vision may also need the creativity of engineers, car manufacturers and our universities. The longer-term cost savings of implementing such a scheme for the delivery of other parts of home care services could be usefully monitored in the pilot sites.

Helping people to get out of their homes is an aspect of service provision that could be developed with other agencies. Local authority social services departments could work with schools or voluntary organisations and early retirees through lifelong learning programmes, to make this relatively low-cost service available. Some people simply want a person to go out with, others need transport. Assistance is often needed to get to local places, not for going on long trips.

Those healthcare services seen as desirable in promoting quality were a prescription service and accessible GPs when people are ill. Clearly this is a matter for negotiation with the PCTs but the local authority social services departments could initiate these developments. A prescription service provided by chemists frees hard-pressed home care staff to do other much-valued tasks such as talking to people or taking them out.

Good health is central to maintaining independence. Being able to get the right treatment remains at one level a matter for science and the transmission of knowledge into health and social care practice. At another it is about access to and organisation of healthcare, health promotion and prevention of ill-health. The value placed on good health by the older people in this study, underpins the importance of providing services which encourage and recognise the skills and abilities of individuals for whom services are being provided.

Quality home care services are, to quote one 90-year-old person, "those which enable you to live at home, which is the most important, because you keep your independence".

This report is organised so that most of the technical information is contained in an appendix. Chapters 1 and 2 set the scene for the research; Chapter 3 contains the main findings relating to older people's views on what quality home care services means to them; Chapter 4 reports our information on quality from ethnic minority groups; Chapter 5 is primarily a toolkit for accessing older people's views and Chapter 6 describes older people's ideas about putting their views on quality into practice so that services in the future will reflect their views and continue to do so.

1
Introductory points: setting and methods

One of the older people who participated in the research project said, "Old age does not come alone". It may come with new needs for assistance and some kinds of health and sensory problems, but it also comes with views. The people who participated in this study made very clear their views about the quality of the services that they would like to see provided in their homes. The importance of listening to the views of service users has been repeatedly stressed in a number of policy documents (DoH, 1989; Hayden and Boaz, 2000).

Aims
The study was designed to achieve three aims:

1. A description of the views of older people on the quality of home care and the priority they attached to the dimensions of quality that they would like to characterise these services.

2. The exploration of ways in which their views can be heard and have an impact on the quality specification of the services delivered.

3. The production of a manual for local authorities on how to access the views of older people on service quality.

Location
Manchester was selected as the study site for a number of reasons. It is a multi-ethnic city faced with the range of problems and opportunities of other major cities in England. As of 1994 there were 46,600 people over the age of 65 and 13,500 people over the age of 80 in Manchester. The City of Manchester Social Services Department (the SSD) purchased home care services on behalf of just under 3,000 of these people.

Manchester is at the bottom of the league for health in England and many Mancunians are struggling against poverty and poor health (Public Health Directorate, 1996). The Jarman (1983) scores (a measure of deprivation commonly used in England) for each of the wards of the City of Manchester show that no Manchester ward has a score higher than the average for England

and Wales. This is represented by zero. Jarman scores at ward level in Manchester run from approximately –60 (indicating low deprivation) to +60 (indicating high deprivation).

Manchester is a multi-ethnic city with Afro-Caribbean, Indian, Pakistani and Chinese as well as Polish, Irish and Jewish communities. The ethnic minority groups recorded in the 1991 Census comprised 12.6% of the total population of the city of Manchester. The national average for England and Wales is 5.9%. Figure 1 shows the ethnic composition of Manchester as recorded in the 1991 census.

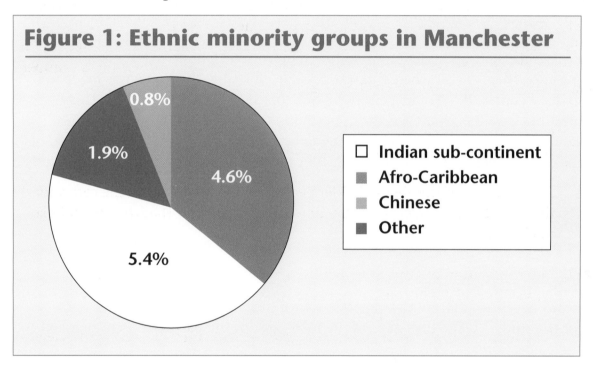

Figure 1: Ethnic minority groups in Manchester

- Indian sub-continent
- Afro-Caribbean
- Chinese
- Other

This study focused on people over the age of 65. The age structure of the ethnic minority groups reported in the Census in Manchester is different from that of the white population. For example, the proportion of ethnic minority residents of pensionable age and over in the 1991 Census was 4.4% compared to 20.5% of the white population. A relatively small proportion of the ethnic minority residents identified in the pie chart was of pensionable age and over in 1991. However there were large numbers of residents in the pre-retirement cohort which means that, in the eight years since the Census, a larger proportion of ethnic minority residents will be approaching or entering the over 65 years cohort.

The principal investigator of this study had previously carried out research in the city, involving the contracting unit in social services. Local knowledge and trust had been built up which it was thought would assist in the current study.

Methods

The population of people for whom home care services were being purchased by the City of Manchester SSD in the Autumn of 1999 was sampled to produce a 10% random sample designed to reflect proportionately the numbers of people under the age of 80 and over the age of 80. A total of 143 people were involved in the study. Of these, 104 were derived from the random sample and 39 were selected from three ethnic minority groups. Details of the sample and the reasons for non-participation in the study are contained in the Appendix.

All 292 people in the sample were sent a letter, which briefly described the project and stated that a member of the research team would contact them to further explain the study. This letter was followed up with telephone contact to arrange for the researchers to visit where this was possible. A visit to the house was made to try to make contact if the older person did not appear to have a telephone. These meetings gave the researchers the opportunity to explain in full what the study would involve if the person was willing to become part of it, and to assure them of the confidentiality of the information they provided. A leaflet explaining the study was left with the person and the opportunity was taken, if they agreed to participate, to complete consent forms. A copy of this form was left with the person and the original was kept in the research files. The older people were given the choice between participating in a focus group or having a home-based interview.

The focus groups

It was necessary to have two separate sets of focus groups to collect the data for the study. At the first stage of the focus groups the participants were asked three questions:

- What services are you getting from any source to enable you to live independently in your home?

- What makes for good quality services at home?

- In an imaginary world when we could have anything we wanted and not pay for it what would make for quality services to maintain your independence at home?

The third question was added during the pilot phase. In the pilot it became apparent that the response to the second question was exceedingly modest and often bound by the participants' awareness that everything was constrained by the reality of money.

In the second set of focus groups, the statements that had been generated in the first focus group as features of quality in home care services were ranked by the participants. They were taught the technique of paired comparisons. This approach works well in any group setting where alternatives must be prioritised. It allows each feature defining quality to be compared with all others. It is a way of gaining a clear view of the priority of items, which appear to have equal merit. Each of the features identified in the first stage focus groups was printed on numbered cards. In the second phase focus groups the participants worked on a one-to-one basis making the comparisons which were recorded on a specially-prepared grid.

Sixth formers from local schools helped to make participants comfortable in all the sessions. In the second stage focus groups they also recorded the results of the paired comparison process for each individual.

The focus groups took place in a number of venues in different parts of the city. The best locations were found in sheltered housing, where we were able to use the communal lounges. Participants at the focus groups sat round tables in stage one. Each of them had their own place name. The discussion was recorded on a flip chart, which most, but not all, of the participants could see, because some that came had sight problems. The scribe responsible for recording the discussion read back to the participants what had been recorded periodically during the course of the meeting. This enabled them to check that she had recorded the information accurately. It also enabled those who could not see, to hear what had been recorded. At all of the focus groups refreshments were provided on arrival and half-way through the one-and-a-half-hour session. Afternoon tea or lunch followed the session, depending on the time of day at which the focus groups occurred. Transport was arranged to enable all of the participants to come to the focus groups. A small number chose to come using transport provided by a friend or member of the family. Where participants wanted a friend or member of the family to accompany them this was agreed, but during the course of the focus groups these people were entertained elsewhere. We took photographs at all the focus groups.

The interviews

Interviews were arranged to suit the convenience of the participants. The interviewees were asked the same three questions as focus group participants. In addition, the interviewees were asked if they would consider the dimensions of quality generated in the focus groups in their area and carry out the paired comparison undertaken by members of the focus groups. Some were willing to do this and some were not.

The data on the desirable quality of home care services came from the 39 participants in the focus groups and from the 64 interviews in people's homes. We have been able to compare whether the different methods of accessing information produce significant differences in the quality characteristics chosen and the ranking given to them. This is a serendipitous aspect of the methodology but of particular relevance to the development of a guide to accessing older people's views about the quality of home services.

The focus groups are an efficient and relatively low cost means of collecting information. They have the advantage of providing a social event for the participants. We came to realise that the groups were, of themselves, a way of building the confidence and capacity of the older people to participate in events in which their voices can be heard. It is our view that in their attitudes to life and their willingness to take risks, the older people who came to these events differed from those we interviewed at home. However, we think that they were surprised by the delight that participation in the meetings gave them. Letters expressed the pleasure they had experienced from being involved in the research project in this way as did the enthusiasm we observed at the time.

Putting ideas into practice

In order to explore ways in which the views expressed could impact on quality specifications and the services delivered, we organised a round-table meeting. This occurred after all of the focus groups and most of the interviews had been completed. Invitations were extended to those who had been at the focus groups and had said they would be interested in continuing to participate in this research. To this same meeting were invited the elected member with cabinet responsibility for social services and other elected members and senior managers from health and social services and the transport and voluntary sector. A total of 10 older people attended this meeting.

At this meeting a brief account of the findings of the research to date was given and some examples of how others elsewhere had shown that it was possible to turn ideas into practice were discussed. Then the group was split into discussion groups and asked to address three questions:

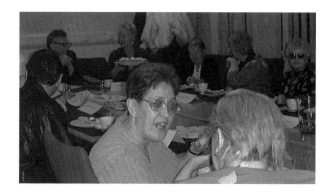

1. How do you ensure that people are heard in setting quality standards?
2. How do you check that the standards are being delivered?
3. What do you need to have in place to make these things happen?

Functional assessment of participants

After much discussion we chose to use the Barthel questionnaire as it appeared to provide, not only a well established, but also a relatively quick means of assessing the capabilities of the participants in the study. It was not possible for these to be completed by the carers or the participants' families. Involving the carers would have been extremely complex as well as violating the commitment to confidentiality, which has been maintained. Many people also lived by themselves. A decision was made to ask the participants to complete the questionnaire themselves. This has resulted in a very small number of questionnaires being returned: 11 from those involved in the focus groups and 43 from those involved in the interviews. This is discussed further in the Appendix.

Chinese and Asian groups

It was thought that one of the difficulties of this study would be accessing the views of older people in some of the city's ethnic minority groups. With the help of members of the Steering Group we were able to meet with members of the Black Consultative Community Care Forum (BCCCF). The Wai Yin Society – a locally-based Chinese organisation, which runs a variety of support activities for members of Manchester's Chinese community – volunteered to run the two-stage focus group model for us. This was done with the help of the research team. Members of the Chinese community, both over and under the age of 80, were invited to participate in the focus groups. The Chinese community conducted the focus groups in Chinese and Haka – a dialect spoken by older members of the Manchester Chinese community. The material was translated into English at the end of first stage so that the cards could be prepared following the identification of the distinct dimensions in the first-stage focus groups. These were then translated into Chinese and the second-stage focus groups followed the model described above.

In the Asian community two separate groups volunteered to find people to participate in the study. In one of these the participants were all male, well educated and under the age of 80. The second community group included both male and female older people who were considerably more disabled than those in first group and more mixed in terms of age. In one of the Asian groups the entire process was conducted in English at the request of group members, which was facilitated by a member of the research team. The other Asian focus group was facilitated by an Urdu-speaking member of the local community assisted by a scribe who wrote up the dimensions of quality in Urdu. These were then translated into English to enable the preparation of the cards for the second-stage focus groups. Individual Urdu or Punjabi volunteers were recruited to carry out the paired comparison rankings in this second-stage focus group.

Neither of these groups were willing to complete the Barthel questionnaires as they regarded them as intrusive. However these four convenience samples give us some information about the views of the Chinese and Asian communities in Manchester.

Contracting for home care services

At the beginning of the study, the Manchester Social Services Contract and Purchasing Unit operated on a spot-purchasing model. Eighteen approved home care service providers were used (providing 60% of services) along with the SSD's own in-house providers. During the course of the study the contracts of the independent purchasers were being renegotiated as the city moved to a cost and volume approach to its purchasing of home care services. During this period local authorities were increasingly focusing on the provision of services to those identified as having the highest and most complex needs.

Analysis of the data

All of the quantitative data was entered into an SPSS file and the coding of the qualitative data was done manually. All the statements in response to the three questions asked in the focus groups were listed. Responses to the two questions designed to focus on older people's views of quality were examined. These were then put into a set of categories according to their focus and then reviewed by the research team to see if anything had been missed. Once these categories had been agreed, all of the statements made in the focus groups and in the interviews were assigned to a category. Thus, each category has a series of descriptors of quality subsumed within it. These operationally-defined categories were used to code both interview and focus group data. A reliability study of the qualitative coding was undertaken on a 10% sample of the qualitative data: 76% agreement was reached on the codes for data relating to people under the age of 80 and 70% agreement for people over the age of 80.

We called these categories 'dimensions of quality' because we wanted a means of indicating that the older people saw services, as multi-faceted, in a multi-dimensional way in effect. We also wanted to suggest that the dimensions have a set of clearly definable and potentially measurable characteristics.

2

Current services

Since 1991 changes have been occurring nationally in the types of services that are delivered to older people living in their own homes. During 1997/98, £1.5 billion were spent by local authorities in Great Britain on the delivery of home care services. Most of this went on provision for older people for whom the expenditure was £1.2 billion in 1996/97 (CIPFA, 1998, 1999). Home care services are big business. In England they are the largest services provided for older people by SSDs. Around 8% of people over the age of 65 receive such a service from local authorities (OPCS, 1996). The tasks involved in the provision of home care have been clearly described (Qureshi et al, 1999; Sinclair et al, 2000). From the perspective of the provider of home care, the tasks to be done for older people are highly varied and the workload is a pressurised one. The delivery of home care services is a complex process involving assessment by a case or care manager, referral from them via the contract and purchasing section of the SSD to the organiser of a contracted service provider and, finally, responsibility for a particular individual is given to the home carer. What the home carer might provide depends primarily on the details in the home care plan, but also, according to Sinclair et al (2000), on what is negotiated between the carer and the person cared for.

Prior to 1991 most home care services were designed to meet basic needs for large numbers of reasonably fit older people unable to cope with some of the tasks of daily living. The services focused largely on the provision of domestic help. This pattern has changed. The policy of community care with its emphasis on maintaining people in their own homes has increased the demands on SSDs. This is especially so in relation to services for very frail older people, who hitherto would have been institutionalised. The growth in the number of very old people, the closure of geriatric wards and the removal of other services previously provided by the NHS have contributed to a shift in the nature of home care services currently provided. Government policy has also caused a shift in the source of home care services so that the growth of the independent sector has been encouraged.

The services designated as 'home care' have shifted greatly in the direction of what is now called personal care as distinct from what used to be called home help. The move from the pre-1991 emphasis on domestic help was encouraged by the Social Services Inspectorate (SSI) publication, *From home help to home care* (SSI, 1987). This change in the range of services to be provided for those identified or assessed as needing home care was followed by the introduction of charges for these services as well as the banding system to determine eligibility for the services themselves.

Manchester SSD is no different from other local authorities in what it is providing under the banner of home care services. Manchester operates both a charging policy and eligibility banding system. Services are commissioned on a half-hour-slot basis and the SSD has a clear set of quality criteria for the provision of services by those from whom it purchases. Home care services are delivered by approximately 30 independent companies and an in-house provider.

Currently there are no nationally agreed quality criteria for the provision of the home care services in all their different manifestations. Under the new 2000 Care Standards Act a set of standards to regulate the provision of home care services will be developed and has been drafted.

Not all home care is provided by agencies under a contract with the local authority SSD. It is still true that much home care is provided by family, friends and neighbours, or purchased independently through the use of the attendance allowance, for example, by the older people themselves.

Types of care

Home care varies. It does so in the types of activities that are provided and the sources of these activities. The older people involved in this research told us about the services they receive and the people who provide them. Even when only considering the services provided by the contracted home carers, the older people in the study identified a large number of different tasks. These included aspects of personal care such as washing, bathing, showering and dressing. They also included more medical or nursing tasks such as providing help to put on elastic stockings, putting ointments on people's backs and buttocks, and changing urostomies. By comparison, somewhat less personal but equally enabling personal services, such as making or changing the bed, helping the older person to dress and preparing meals for them, were also identified as part of the services being delivered. Additionally, shopping tasks were carried out, as well as the collection of pensions and payment of bills. A number of older people interpreted home care to mean the aids and adaptations which have been provided to make it possible for them to live independently in their homes. These included adaptations to their baths and the provision of walk-in showers and stair-lifts for example. The provision of panic buttons and pendants linked to telephone call centres were also seen as part of the home care service, along with special cutlery and the availability of a ring-and-ride service which enables older people to get themselves about. In addition to all of these services, cleaning services, vacuuming and dusting and washing still played a part in the services delivered in Manchester to older people in their homes.

Family and neighbours

Family and neighbours were identified as sources of help with shopping – in particular being taken out shopping – assistance with the garden and the cleaning of windows. In some instances family members and neighbours were described as 'popping in' to check that everything is OK but went beyond this activity to offer specific help in putting people to bed, getting them up, getting their pension and papers and in taking them to hospital appointments. The provision of a prescription service by some chemists was used by some of the people in this study.

Private arrangements

A number of the older people in this study had made their own arrangements for home care services. These focused largely around the provision of window cleaners and gardeners. Some had their own private cleaners and arrangements to enable the ironing to be done. A small number had made private arrangements for aids and adaptations such as a shower, a stair-lift or alarms to be fitted to their homes.

The home care services provided in Manchester for the older people in this study are clearly very varied. We have attempted to summarise the range of activities that they experience as home care in the pie charts below. When asked about the home services they receive the older people came up with many examples. We grouped these into distinct categories. Sometimes the older people would give several examples of the same category of service and each one of these was counted as an example of that category. The older people's perceptions of what they currently receive are presented in Figures 2 and 3. The percentages reflect the number of times an example of a type of service was mentioned.

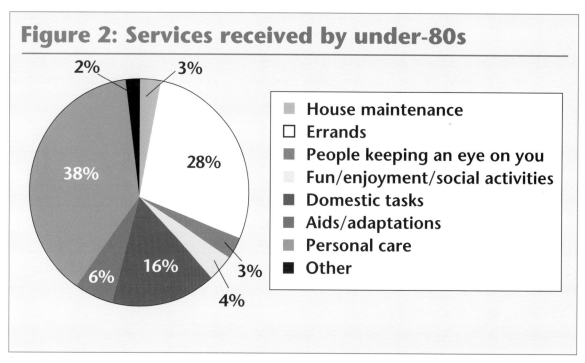

Figure 2: Services received by under-80s

- House maintenance
- Errands
- People keeping an eye on you
- Fun/enjoyment/social activities
- Domestic tasks
- Aids/adaptations
- Personal care
- Other

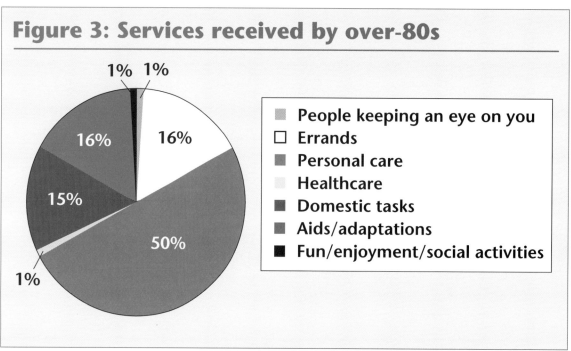

Figure 3: Services received by over-80s

- People keeping an eye on you
- Errands
- Personal care
- Healthcare
- Domestic tasks
- Aids/adaptations
- Fun/enjoyment/social activities

The information provided in these pie charts provides a picture of the service context in which this study took place. The next chapter considers the views of older people in Manchester about the qualities they would like to see in the services that arrive, one way or another, to their homes to enable them to live there independently.

3
Older people's views on home care services

A small number of other studies have explored older people's views of service quality. Henwood et al (1998), using a convenience sample, tried to identify the features of service delivery that mattered most to service users and their carers. Attributes such as staff reliability, continuity of care and of staff, kindness and cheerfulness, competence in undertaking tasks and flexibility responding to change in need, knowledge of the service user and availability of clear information about services were identified as important in that study.

A larger study carried out in the United States (Woodruff and Appelbaum, 1996) provided similar evidence that stressed the importance placed on services which enable older people to maintain control. They also identified the importance, for older people, of services being reliable, delivered competently and being responsive to their needs. However, neither of these studies attempted to identify the *priority* of these aspects of quality. In a Swedish study, Edelbalk et al (1995) did explore the relative importance attached to quality characteristics of home care services. Their study identified five major quality dimensions at a general level: influence and control, personal relationships, continuity, availability, time and suitability of the home help. Edelbalk and his colleagues (1995) used the multi-attribute utility technology technique to rank the relative importance that older people attach to valued characteristics that the researchers had derived from earlier work. In our study, the statements made by the older people themselves about what a quality home care service would be are those which were used in the paired comparison ranking to determine the relative importance of each attribute of quality. We have not been able to find any other study in the literature which does this.

Most of the studies of user satisfaction, including the Best Value studies which are now undertaken by local authorities, indicate high levels of satisfaction with the services provided (see for example, Godfrey et al, 2000).

In this chapter the views of the people who came to focus groups are reported first, then the views of those interviewed in their own homes are reported. Finally, we summarise the priority the older people gave to the dimensions of quality that they identified as contributing to a high quality home care service.

Dimensions of quality home care services raised by people aged under and over the age of 80

In this study when older people talk about the quality of home care services they talk about both their content and the way in which they are provided. They do not differentiate between the 'what' and the 'how' of services. They also do not only talk about what comes into their homes but what enables them to get out. It is as if their view of home care is rounded so that what happens in your home and what you experience there is also affected by what you do and experience outside it. This is not how home care providers think of home care, nor how services are themselves connected or constructed. When asked, 'What would make for good quality home care services?', many of the issues the older people raised are not traditionally seen as part of home care services at all. However, these things influence the way they live and their views on the quality of the services that they would like delivered to their homes. We have included what was said about these issues, since they were raised in the context of a discussion about home care services.

As far as possible we have used the words of the older people themselves. We felt that too much reorganisation would conceal rather than reveal what they told us. Thus, in this chapter there are a series of lists and quotations which are grouped into major categories (see the Appendix for details of the methods). We refer to these categories as the 'dimensions of care'. To avoid long lists and repetition of descriptors we have condensed some of the responses. People both under and over the age of 80 who came to our focus groups or were interviewed in their own homes referred to features of home care which could be classified into one of six categories or dimensions of home care. These are:

1. What carers do.

2. How carers are organised.

3. Aids and adaptations.

4. Going out.

5. Transport.

6. Improvements in health services.

In addition, people under the age of 80 identified the provision of opportunities to have some company, feeling safe and having more money, as dimensions of a good quality home care service. Those over the age of 80 spoke of the importance of keeping their mind occupied, and the provision of robots as part of provision in a quality home care service. Under each of the six dimensions, those ideals common to both groups are described first, followed by those issues which were age specific.

What carers do

People both under and over the age of 80 identified a good quality service as one in which carers:

- help with housework to keep the house clean, vacuuming, polishing, high shelves, cleaning the brass, wash the paint work down, keep your standards about how your home should look;

- change your bed and make beds properly;

- help with odd jobs around the house;

- look after the garden;

- help with decorating;

- help with spring cleaning;

- help with washing large items of laundry;

- clean the insides of windows;

- take washing to the launderette;

- do the ironing;

- take you out shopping so you can see what you are buying;

- help with little things such as laces, stockings, socks, trousers;

- provide physical support to take you out so you are not afraid of falling;

- provide a bathing service and cut fingernails;

- deliver fresh food for people to cook;

- can get a prescription for you;

- provide food and supplies when you are ill;

- do the banking and letter posting;

- talk to you about your problems;

- treat you with respect;

- have a nice friendly smile;

- are gentle and kind.

All of these describe the tasks and personal attributes that carers would provide in a quality home care service. Essential elements are the provision of help with domestic tasks, personal care and errands. Also central is emotional support and befriending. The personal characteristics of carers as they carry out valued tasks, contribute to the quality of the service that people want. Other studies have identified the importance clients place on these attributes of home care services (Edelbalk et al, 1995).

The concern with keeping things clean was described by one participant under the age of 80 as, "Help with cleaning to keep it how you want it". Another participant, who was over the age of 80, requested, "Glasses shining; windows you can see through and curtains clean, and dusting and vacuuming under as well as around things".

Keeping things clean appears to be very important in people's lives. The immediate environment in which people spend much of their life needs to be controlled and reflect this, even if they are crumbling within it:

"Keeping things like you used to." (Woman, over 80)

"Help with the tops and bottoms of cupboards and with high shelves." (Woman, over 80)

"The curtains and windows need to be done and you're there, sitting looking at them." (Woman, over 80)

The importance of domestic help has also been noted in other studies (Challis and Davies, 1986; Godfrey et al, 2000), however, this contrasts markedly with the SSI recommendations that services should focus on the provision of personal social care.

From the perspective of the older people in this study, the level of domestic help required to make a quality service was not necessarily great. For example, one focus group member said: "A little help with housework – 'hoovering' especially – would help".

There was much concern with maintaining the standards of cleanliness that they had obtained earlier in their lives:

> "If you haven't got a family, who's going to do your windows, work surfaces, dusting and polishing if you can't?" (Woman, under 80)

> "Looking at dirty curtains is very depressing, but I can't reach to take them down." (Woman, under 80)

Untended bushes in the garden can cut out light, as one man, under 80, commented: "If the privets were cut I could see out of the windows".

It appears as if the older people wish to control their immediate environment and ensure that it is kept the way it was. The care of their home is a reflection of them and their pride in who they are; it is also what they see each day. It is something they want to maintain even if they cannot do it but, as one participant put it, that they "want to be able to do".

Getting help with personal care and errands should also be part of a quality service. One man over the age of 80 was quite specific in saying that he wanted "a bathing service, three or four times a week at least". We were told by a woman under 80 that "shoppers aren't allowed to get the prescriptions, you need someone to do this", if a quality service is to be provided.

The way in which the carers carry out their work is clearly important: gentleness, respect and cheerfulness are valued:

> "I want to be treated with respect, not, 'I'll just pop you into bed'. You should have the right to say the earliest you want to go to bed." (Woman, under 80, unable to walk)

"[You need] a carer who treats you with respect so that you are able to say thank you to the carer." (Woman, aged 84)

"People who have been carers in their lives are entitled to gentle handling." (Woman, aged 84, who is blind)

Organisation of carers
A good quality service is one in which:

- you have your entitlement in writing so you know what the limits are;

- communication is improved between clients, carers and care managers;

- if a stranger comes instead of our regular carer you are told who is coming for safety reasons;

- there is better management of services and carers are managed more efficiently;

- you are able to rely on what the carer does and when (for example, what time s/he will be back with the shopping);

- the office informs you when things will be done or tells you that someone will be late;

- there is more coordination between the people who come out to help and the organisation;

- the service is monitored (to include spot checks on carers);

- there is one manager who knows about you and to whom you can have access if you need to get something done;

- time is not wasted by duplication of services;

- there is a book to record payments in rather than the current flimsy bits of paper;

- carers stay for their allocated time;

- carers remain for enough time to build up a relationship;

- carers have proper cover so that they are not forced to take on extra work without the time to do it;

- organisers listen to people's needs and respond to them;

- carers do what you ask them to without complaining or saying that they are not allowed;

- carers ask you what you want them to do and work with you, rather than do what someone else has told them to do, and will negotiate over services that the client wants (for which they would pay more if necessary);

- organisers do not tell the carers one story and the clients another, nor treat clients like children and 'unwanted parcels';

- there is good basic training for carers in how to care, how to clean and in the emotional aspects of caring;

- there is a standard set for carers;

- carers come more often than once a week;

- office-based staff know about you and your needs.

Key elements of this dimension are the provision of information about the service, its continuity and reliability. A quality service is also one which is flexible, so that it can be responsive and sensitive to individuals. Older people also thought that the carers' ability to enhance the quality of the things they do for people would be increased if they were given further training. Additionally, the service should be monitored to see that these features, and others of a quality service, are in place.

Having your entitlement in writing would mean that "you know what the limits are, and they [the carers] wouldn't say I can't do that" (Man, under 80).

> "An entitlement in writing would save unpleasantness. So you can ask them to do what you want them to do and they will do it without moaning. For example windows, changing your curtains, prescriptions. They won't say we are not allowed." (Woman, under 80)

Many times we heard people talk about the need for someone to inform them if a new person was coming to their house. It is quite frightening when you do not know who is coming to your house and you are blind or partially sighted. As one lady put it, a quality service would be one where those who came to your house were "not strangers coming instead of regular carers. We need some form of identity; we need to know who is coming for safety" (Woman from the under-80s focus group). This view was echoed in an over-80s focus group by someone who said that what is needed is:

> "Carers who know you and know where to come, not thirty different people! A regular person and somebody to let you know if someone different is coming and if it is a stranger." (Woman, aged 90)

There are other advantages to having the same person provide your care. As one person, aged 84, said: "You don't have to tell them over and over; they know what to do and where things are. A trusting relationship is built up and they don't have to be watched".

Older people still have their own lives to live, so "knowing that the carer is coming at a particular time so that you can organise around it" enables them to continue to control their own lives rather than let the help they get take over. If a carer is doing shopping it is important that they "come back when they say they will", and it is important for the "office to inform you when things will be done and when someone will be late".

Many comments were made about the need for a quality service to be one which is flexible and responsive to people's needs. Illustrative of this are two comments:

> "The carer [should] work with you and say, 'What would you like me to do?', even just once a month." (Woman, aged 70)

> "You need the help to work with you, it's always doing what someone else tells them to do. Two or three hours, it would be nice if they said, 'What would you like me to do?' – just once a month for the cupboards or bit of polishing. We need one boss who knows about you and you can have access to them. Knowing somebody who can help you get something done." (Woman, aged 84)

In such a service carers would be helped by training and the improved planning of the service so that "they had time to make a bed, not just straighten it, and they knew how to do it". Another person said that in a quality service there would be "less wasted time because of badly-planned journeys between clients. Instead there would be neighbourhood workers who don't waste time driving about". All carers would have "good basic training in how to care, how to clean and the emotional aspects".

Older people understood that the service was made up of different parts and said:

> "More co-ordination is needed between people who come out to help and the organisation. You need organisers who listen to people's needs and respond to them." (Man, aged 85)

> "We should not be wasting time and help by duplication of services. Better management of services is needed."

A responsive service would be monitored:

> "Social services should come at least twice a year to check that you are happy with the services. Social services are too remote." (Woman, aged 83)

A quality service is one where:

> "[The carer] comes at agreed times, their work is checked from time to time giving you the opportunity to complain or approve. Giving you a voice this way. Flexible in what they will do, the carers. Responsive to needs without being asked, for example, they'll clean windows when the window cleaner is not available. The opportunity to pay for extra work when needed. Personal negotiation because you know the person." (Woman from over-80s focus group)

Aids and adaptations
A good quality service is one in which:

- your accommodation is appropriate;

- there is a means of communicating with people at your front door if your flat is upstairs;

- there is a stair-lift or banisters;

- you have a pendant panic alarm in case you fall, linked to a telephone and call centre;

- you have a shower with easy access or some way of getting out of the bath easily;

- a reclining chair is available;

- there are cheaper rental phones, with low-user tariffs for emergency-only users;

- buildings have doors wide enough for wheelchairs;

- there is an easier way of transporting medical oxygen supplies;

- there are more seats between shops and in shops

- there are taps with handles that make it easy to turn them off;

- there are shopping trolleys like four-wheeled prams (such as those provided by Tescos which are designed to be easier to push).

The key distinction in what older people identified in this dimension of home care services is that some related to their homes and others to help that could be provided in the world outside to enable them to get about. In the former group were the emergency pendants which were much valued by those who had them, but were not universally known about. Telephones are not usually thought of as aids or adaptations, however, as one man put it, "the 'phone is a lifeline for housebound people, but there should be lower tariffs, not £60 per call" (this man would use his telephone in emergencies – this is what he meant by a lifeline – the annual rental seemed to him exorbitant for such, hopefully, infrequent calls). Participants also requested:

> "An intercom with a camera so that you can identify visitors." (Woman from over-80s group)

> "An intercom without the door opening." (Woman from under-80s group)

These would promote a sense of security. A stair-lift or an easily-accessible shower would enable more independence for some, as would somewhere to sit when outside their own home.

Getting out

A good quality service is one in which:

- you can get out and meet people;

- there are people to go out with;

- there are day centres where various services as well as company are on offer;

- you can go shopping and see what you are getting;

- there are affordable clubs that you can go to;

- you have a garden to sit out in;

- there is a respite home for a complete change but which is not full of people with dementia;

- you can get a holiday with no single supplement charge;

- there is a day-trip service that caters for wheelchairs that you can telephone and book;

- you can have a day out that someone organises.

Key issues here relate to enabling people to get out for a number of different purposes. As one man put it: "A change of scenery and a trip out makes you feel good". Another described getting out as "being like therapy – you're lifted up by going out, it takes the depression off you". Going out is inextricably linked to transport and company, and for most people getting out is both easier and more pleasurable if someone else is there to help. For some older people, other people's assistance in getting out is essential not just an added pleasure. A woman in an under-80s focus group suggested an "adopt a granny or grandpa scheme would be good. Someone to go out with to hold onto to get over this fear of falling". Going out promotes choice and independence. To this end "help with going out so you can shop for yourself, choose for yourself, not have someone else's decisions" would promote a quality service. The benefits of getting out are seen as connecting people with the world and extending and enriching life. Provision of transport plays an important part in this.

Transport

A good quality service is one in which:

- there is affordable and accessible transport;

- there is transport to a range of destinations;

- buses do not jolt so you can have confidence when you get onto a bus;

- there is a way of getting to and from bus stops and in and out of shops;

- subsidised transport is available to go anywhere;

- there is a transport service for hospital appointments;

- there is transport to get to see family in different parts of the country;

- there is space for your motorised chair;

- there are mini-bus agencies which are good;

- there are low-floor buses which are level with the kerb and have space for wheelchairs, so that you can take advantage of having a bus pass;

- there is a ring-and-ride service;

- you can use an electric buggy with safe lanes to drive on which are free from traffic; which would mean that you could do more for yourself such as shopping and taking the dog out;

- you can have a moped or bike, and somewhere safe to store it;

- there is a means of transferring from wheelchair to scooter;

- pavements and roads are made safe for wheelchairs;

- there is a car available for personal use.

What the older people had to say about transport is not often seen as part of home care services however, they raised these matters in the focus groups as relevant to home care services. From their perspective transport is a part of what made for good quality home care services. Transport plays a significant role in being able to get out: a ring-and-ride service can get you to a coach station to enable you to go on longer trips or more simply to the shops, friends or a hospital. Feeling safe and secure on these vehicles is as important as their being affordable and accessible:

> "[We need] stable transport that is not so frightening. You need to feel normal, so you need to be able to use public transport." (Woman, aged 86)

> "Pavements and roads made safe for wheelchairs", and buses modified so that "they are level with the curb and have space for wheelchairs." (Man, under 80)

In one way it is transport that can pull together all aspects of quality. The man who said that, in an imaginary world, "there would be electric buggies and dedicated lanes for them on the roads, and places to keep them safe", went on to point out that if this existed he could get out himself; he could shop for food, visit others who were housebound and do their shopping for them, and keep himself cheerful.

Improvements in health services
A good quality service is one in which:

- there is a comprehensive health service and older people are not discriminated against; doctors investigate as far as they can;

- doctors will come and see you and have access to technology;

- there is enough money in the system to provide 24-hour cover;

- when you are ill you can rely on the doctor doing what he promises;

- the doctor/chemist/prescription service is consistently available so that those who want to use it can access it at any time;

- doctors should explain what is wrong so that you can understand;

- you can see a doctor rather than just get repeat prescriptions;

- you can see a doctor for a general medical check up.

The key issues here were around access to medical services and the availability of a prescription service:

> "You need help when you are ill. You need to be able to rely on people for support, especially the doctor doing what he says he will." (Man, under 80)

> "A doctor who will come out and not just prescribe, and you can go and see the doctor for a check up." (Man, over 80)

People both under and over the age of 80 spoke of the importance of good health in generating a good quality of life for themselves. Health services are one contributor to this. The importance of older people in the provision of their services is often overlooked – they are the central actors in the picture. Being in good health is a necessary prerequisite to maintaining independence.

Both groups were keen to retain their existing range of services, which were described in Chapter 2, and participants were unequivocal in their view that the services they currently received should be maintained. They referred to examples of the wide range of services described in Chapter 2, as well as to the adaptations and aids provided to keep them in their own homes and maintain their independence. As several put it: "Keep what you've got: I couldn't exist without my carer".

Others commented on the aids they had been provided with. For example a man said, "I couldn't exist without my shower".

However, their desire to keep what they already had in the way of home care services did not stop them from identifying what quality in home care and other related services meant to them.

Other characteristics of quality services specific to people under the age of 80

People under the age of 80 also identified three other dimensions of a quality home care service. These were company, feeling safe and money.

Company

For people under the age of 80 a good quality service is one in which:

- you can get out and meet people;

- there is someone to go out for a meal with;

- you are able to travel to see grandchildren and other family members;

- there is someone to talk to every day;

- neighbours take time for people and take notice;

- you have visitors who come for a chat or for a walk;

- in sheltered housing there is someone to organise coffee mornings, cinema shows and other events;

- you can meet younger people who are not set in their ways;

- there is someone to share problems, fears and worries with; someone to confide in;

- you are able to see people passing by;

- there is a warden who can organise events to bring people together.

The companionship people saw as important in providing quality was as much about dealing with loneliness as it was about literally and figuratively getting out of their home, escaping the proverbial four walls and re-expanding their worlds:

> "Talking to people gets rid of some of your worries, it takes you out of yourself." (Man, under 80)

> "Someone to talk to lightens the load and shares your problems, both for you and for them." (Woman, under 80)

> "Having someone to come in and have chat with, go out with [would] make my day." (Woman, under 80)

For one man, provision of a quality service, in terms of this service dimension, would be to enable him to "get out once or twice a week, daily if possible".

People under the age of 80 appeared to view company as important as getting jobs around the house done, personal care, house maintenance and being treated respectfully, with cheerfulness and flexibility. Sinclair et al (2000) noted how carers themselves are aware of this aspect of the care they provide, notwithstanding the task-oriented nature of their jobs and the half-hour slots (or multiples of these) allocated for their time with the clients.

In the focus groups for people under 80, feeling safe and money issues were also raised as attributes of what is perhaps better described as quality of life issues. They are included in this report because they are about services and because they were raised by clients in the context of home care services.

Feeling safe

A good quality service is one in which:

- pavements and roads are made safe for wheelchairs;

- there is no fear of break-ins or discarded needles;

- police take notice of what you say;

- the postperson pushes letters through the letterbox – otherwise people can take them out.

Older people in this age group took the view that improvements in the world outside their homes could enhance their home care and their sense of security in their homes.

Money

A good quality service is one in which:

- you can get a free dog licence;

- you can have a free TV licence;

- you do not have to pay for the extra help needed when you are ill;

- you have more money.

Other characteristics of quality services specific to people over the age of 80

People over the age of 80 saw things that would keep their mind occupied and the provision of robots as important elements of a quality home care service. An illustration of the former was the idea that "books, jigsaws to swap with friends are available" (woman, over 80). The robots were seen as a means of getting some practical tasks done:

> "[They would] accompany you to the library, shops and carry things for you." (Woman, over 80)

> "They would do things around the house including making a cup of tea for you." (Man, over 80)

The views of people at home under and over the age of 80

The home-based interviews generated no new dimensions of quality but they gave people in their own homes the opportunity to express their views. Interviewees made similar comments about what would generate improved quality in their home care services. There was, as in the focus groups, much appreciation for services currently being provided:

> "I am very thankful for such people, as home carers are what makes it possible for people to live at home, which is the most important thing because you keep your independence." (Man, aged 90)

However, the quality of services provided by carers would be promoted by being able to give some more help:

> "A shower every day, not just two times per week, would be nice." (Man, over 80)

> "The carer being able to collect medication from the chemist." (Woman, under 80)

Wardens of sheltered accommodation also came in for much praise:

> "She listens to me, it really makes a difference, just a little chat." (Woman, over 80)

Provision of cleaning would promote a quality service:

> "All older people should have someone clean their house." (Man, over 80)

In relation to the organisation of services one person said that "their complaint resulted in the service not coming". Another person expressed a commonly-held view: "When the carer doesn't come on time I get panicky".

"There are two choices, you have it [the service] or you don't." (Man, aged 80)

"Lack of continuity means you can't build a relationship and they don't know where things are." (Woman, over 80)

The need to check and monitor was clearly illustrated in the extreme case of one man who told us, "The carer did not arrive and I had to 'phone at 11 pm and ask to be put to bed". As in the focus groups, the interviewees requested a list so that people know what carers can and cannot do and this was seen as part of a quality service. Allegedly one carer had told a client that the s/he "was only allowed to go down one road to do the shopping".

These comments clearly suggest that developing a quality service means doing things differently.

Some helpful suggestions and new ideas about how to improve the organisation of services were made which had not been suggested in the focus groups. One was the facility to pay for services using direct debit, "so you didn't have to worry about having the money". The perceived limitations about where the carers were allowed to do shopping resulted in one interviewee employing someone to shop for her, "because the local shop doesn't stock the kind of food I can eat...". She suggested, "Couldn't Safeway give me a list of what it stocks so that I can widen my choice of food and avoid monotony?". Providing carers with bicycles or company cars was another suggestion made by a man (aged 91) whose carers were often late or replaced by another because, as he put it, "they drove old bangers".

Aids and adaptations were also seen as part of a quality service. One man said that a motorised wheelchair would be seen as a mark of a quality service, so that "my wife and I could go walking in the woods and over the fields like we used to". Another man said, "A shower would make me a very happy person".

Similar comments were made on the improvements needed in healthcare services. As in the focus groups, interviewees discussed aspects of the quality of their life which go beyond what is usually thought of as home care. Among the issues they raised were: money – "just a bit more of it"; and feeling secure – "free from racist attacks", as one interviewee put it.

Their comments on the importance of getting out and transport were no different from their peers who came to the focus groups.

In relation to company one lady said, "I would like someone to come in the evening, particularly in the winter. Friends are unwilling to visit in the evening".

Priorities

Some of the interviewees (66%) completed the ranking of the descriptors of quality generated in the focus groups held in their part of the city.

When we compare the ranking of the descriptions of quality in home care services generated in the focus groups and ranked by the group participants and the interviewees, there is overlap in their top ten rankings. Comparing the ratings of people over and under the age of 80 does show that they assess the relative importance of six dimensions differently; however, both groups place the following dimensions at the top of their lists:

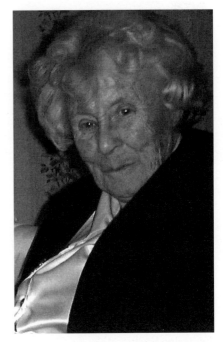

- What carers do

- Getting out

- How carers are organised

- Aids and adaptations

- Transport

- Improvements in health services.

The people under the age of 80 also included:

- Company.

Local authorities and independent service providers could take action to change things and promote quality in home care services in terms of what carers do, the organisation of the services and aids and adaptations. Helping people get out and about would need their input as well as that of other agencies such as transport, highways, and perhaps schools or young people's services. It is noteworthy that it would require the health service, as well as transport services and the police to make changes that would address the other highly rated attributes.

4

Views on quality of home care services from three minority ethnic groups

Following discussion with the local Steering Group and the Advisory Group to the project, we decided that we were unlikely to get many of the people from the minority ethnic groups identified in the 1991 Census to come to the focus groups or be interviewed. It was argued that many minority ethnic groups did not use services provided or purchased by Manchester SSD. It was suggested that they would not relate to or understand the white middle-class researchers involved in the project. We therefore made attempts to find other ways of hearing their voices. The SSD had established a Black Consultative Community Care Forum (BCCCF) and members of this group sat on the local Steering Group to the project. The research team was invited to meet with them and other BCCCF members. Several minority ethnic groups were then approached: the Wai Yin Chinese Women's Society, the Elderly Asian Development Group and the Longsight/Moss Side Community Project offered to help with the research and

to try out the focus group model.

In our efforts to hear the voices of people from these communities we learned a considerable amount. This learning was not restricted to hearing what people from different communities had to say about the desirable qualities of good quality home care services, but extended to methodological issues about accessing such information.

First, each group is introduced and their views on home care services and the qualities they would like to see are outlined. We then make some brief observations about the issues of working with the other communities and link this with other literature about such matters.

Wai Yin Chinese Women's Society

This society was established in 1988 by a group of dedicated and community-minded Chinese women. These women felt that the views and needs of Chinese women were not being represented in Manchester, and that Chinese women were discriminated against both by British society and their own community and families. The Wai Yin Chinese Women's Society was re-launched in March of 2000 and has developed a wide range of projects. Its management committee members are still all women. The society gained funding from the Mental Health Social Care Partnership and obtained a second round of funding from the National Lottery Charities Board. It also receives funding from the SSD.

Of particular relevance to this research is the society's 'elderly project' which aims to provide a social club setting; information and advice; organised cultural and social programmes and increased social interaction. Its target group is Chinese women and men above the age of 60. Among other things, it provides a luncheon club four days a week, current affairs information through news reports, physical exercise suitable for older people, talks on health and related issues aimed specifically at older Chinese people, interpretation, translation, letter reading, form filling and related services. It also organises trips to places of interest. The society and the luncheon club are located in the middle of Manchester's Chinatown. The director and her colleagues thought that members of the luncheon club would be interested in participating in the research project.

Methods

It was agreed that the data collection process would follow that used in the main study. The Chinese team was briefed in a number of meetings about the running of the focus groups. Two focus groups were arranged, each with 10 older people – one for people under the age of 80 and one for people over the age of 80. The group for people over the age of 80 was facilitated in the morning prior to lunch. This group joined the other group of people under the age of 80 for lunch and then left. Mr Ho then facilitated a second focus group for 10 people under the age of 80. Both focus groups were conducted in Cantonese and Haka. At the request of the staff of the Wai Yin Society a member of the research team remained throughout the two focus groups and the lunch. The discussion was recorded in Mandarin Chinese. All the members of the staff of the Wai Yin Chinese Women's Society who assisted in the two focus groups were known to the luncheon club members.

Characteristics of the two groups

Older Chinese people generally live close to the centre of Manchester and 90% of the luncheon club members live within five miles of the city centre. Most of them live in flats built by different housing associations. According to the society's coordinator, most of them knew of the existence of care services. 80% of the luncheon club members are female and 20% are male and these proportions are represented in the composition of the focus groups. A total of 90% of the luncheon club members are between the ages of 65 and 80, and only 10% are over the age of 80. The oldest member of the luncheon club is 95 years old.

The members of the focus groups were categorised by Wai Yin staff using their own categories. These are: healthy independent (probably not thinking about using care services yet); health condition deteriorating (using care services or will need some forms of care soon); living with the family (getting help from family members); or living in residential homes (totally dependent). The distribution of these categories are given below in Figure 4.

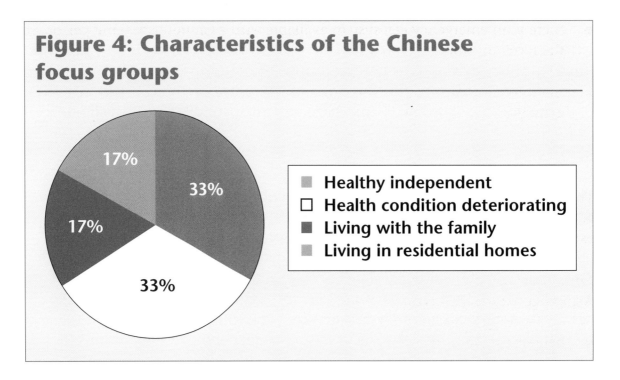

Figure 4: Characteristics of the Chinese focus groups

- Healthy independent
- Health condition deteriorating
- Living with the family
- Living in residential homes

A number of participants from the Wai Yin focus groups completed the Barthel questionnaires. The Barthel scores show that the mean score was 19.38 with a standard deviation of 0.74. The maximum score on this measure, reflecting full independence, is 20, this shows the Chinese group to be very independent.

People under 80: services currently being used

Some members of this group had never heard of home care services and were looking after themselves. Others used a paid service getting an hour a week, and others were looked after by their spouses.

People under 80: Chinese views on the dimensions of good quality home care services

This group came up with 28 aspects of quality. These have been grouped within the categories developed in the initial part of the study. It was possible to group most of the features in this way, however, there was an additional set that can only be described as the Chinese dimension.

The Chinese dimension

A good quality service was defined as one in which:

- there are Chinese interpreters in hospitals and with doctors;

- there is an emergency call system available with a Chinese-speaking person at the receiving end;

- there is a more spacious Chinese day centre with ease of access and various activities;

- there are carers who speak English and Chinese.

The other dimensions they outlined were: organisation of services, aids and adaptations, better health services and money. These are listed below with examples of the descriptors given by this group.

Organisation of services

A good quality service is one in which:

- helpers are trained;

- training includes confidentiality, social work and DIY skills;

- services are planned around older people's needs, living habits and medical requirements.

Aids and adaptations

A good quality service is one in which:

- showers and curtains are fitted in your house free of charge.

Improvements in health services

A good quality service is one in which:

- medical standards are improved, especially in casualty.

Money

A good quality services is one in which:

- the TV licence fee is waived;

- water rates are waived.

People over 80: services currently being used

As with the younger group, there were some people who had never heard of home care services and were looking after all aspects of daily living themselves. There were also people paying an hourly charge for a cleaning service and others who were getting help from members of their family. There was a very strong view in this group that "I would rather die than live in an aged home", but this was matched by the view that "having a Chinese aged home where diet, communication and language posed no problems at all" might make living somewhere other than in your own home more tolerable. Views about neighbours as sources of help were mixed. It was said that "some are excellent", but others said: "There is no communication between the neighbours; a few elderly people died in their room and this was only discovered after several days".

People over 80: Chinese views on the dimensions of good quality home care services

This group came up with 18 descriptions of a quality service which had a strong Chinese focus. Six of the 18 examples were in the Chinese dimension; the others fell into categories already developed: the organisation of services, aids and adaptations, money and transport.

The Chinese dimension

A good quality service is one in which:

- there are Chinese interpreters at clinics;

- there are Chinese wardens, especially at night;

- there are Chinese speakers to read letters, fill out forms;

- there is transport to Chinese day centres;

- there is a Chinese older people's home;

- there is a Chinese day centre;

- there are Chinese and Haka speaking carers.

The other dimensions, with examples of the descriptors they gave, are as follows.

Organisation of services

A good quality service is one in which:

- the carers are trained.

Aids and adaptations

A good quality service is one in which:

- old furniture is removed.

Transport

A good quality service is one in which:

- transport is arranged between home and clinic.

Money

A good quality service is one in which:

- services for people over the age of 70 are free.

The Elderly Asian Development Group

This group is one of a number of groups within the Asian community in Manchester. There are some disagreements among members of this community in the city, which has led to a proliferation of Pakistani organisations.

The Elderly Asian Development Group caters for older members of the community. It has a newspaper written in both English and Urdu which is produced every month. The group distributes 500 copies of the magazine via mosques and libraries. Its editor is a lawyer and translates the medical and other information from English into Urdu. A forum is also organised on a monthly basis. This meets in a number of different places because of the difficulty of finding locations which are sympathetic to the dietary needs of the group and the fact that they hold their meetings on a Sunday afternoon. The organisation is supported by a grant from the health authority.

Ten male members of this organisation agreed to become involved in the research. At an initial meeting there was some clear hostility to the project and a number of issues were raised. It was stated that no one knew what home care was and that there was a need for leaflets in Urdu and Punjabi to be distributed to mosques to inform people of their entitlements. It was pointed out that in India and Pakistan, many services to support older members of the family have to be purchased. It is also regarded that certain tasks should only be done by members of low level castes, for example, cutting hair and dealing with soiled clothing.

Characteristics of the group

All of the members of the group were under the age of 80. All of them spoke in English. They asked that the focus groups at both stages be conducted in English. They did not provide any completed Barthel questionnaires as they saw these as intrusive. All of them were able to walk, one with some difficulty. We have no other information about the individual characteristics of the members of this group.

Services currently being used

This group was generally unaware that there were home care services. They commented on the lack of assistance of any kind that they received. In some cases the men's families did washing, shopping, collecting pensions and cooking, and some had experience of a district nurse visiting following a hospital episode. They made the point that it was hard for their families to assist them because they had to take time off from their work or their studies. It was clearly the view of every member of the group that they received nothing from social services and any support that was available came only from their families. The group also said that they did not know where to go to buy services. One person said: "To qualify for a service you have to be a dead person because they make it so difficult to get". The basis for this observation was the completion of forms which this man thought were so complicated that half-way through he realised he did not qualify. Another person said:

> "You have to be locked into poverty and not have your children helping you because they will count against you. They, the social services, value the services of children so you deprive yourself of services if your family help you."

The group maintained that the help available focused on manpower rather than on aids (such as a stair-lift) which could make a person more independent.

Asian views on the dimensions of good quality home care services

This group came up with 25 different features of what a quality service would be to them. These features largely fell into the dimensions generated by this age group in the main study. In their top ten ranked dimensions were those relating to the organisation of services and the provision of aids and adaptations. There was a different dimension specific to this group which related to their families: they wanted them to be to rewarded for their help to their parents and assisted to provide that help in other ways.

The Asian dimension
A good quality service is one in which:

- families are rewarded financially for helping their older relatives;

- jobs for children are brought closer to their family home.

The other dimensions, with examples of the descriptors they gave, are as follows.

Organisation of services
A good quality service is one in which:

- the service is delivered in time and when needed;

- accessing the service does not require intrusive procedures;

- assessment is user friendly and focuses on granting help, not denying people's needs;

- there is easy and quick access to essential services;

- services help without humiliating.

Aids and adaptations

A good quality service is one in which:

- the focus is on providing aids and adaptations which promote independence.

They also discussed wider quality of life issues in the context of home care services. They ranked highly the need to be financially and physically independent so that there was, as they put it, "no need to ask for help".

The Longsight/Moss Side Community Project

Funding from the SSD supports this community project which provides a variety of different activities, including support services for older people and training for staff. The project is also trying to develop an awareness within the community of what home care services could provide. Muslim and Hindu care workers have been trained but these people are now being treated as low caste people in both the Indian and Pakistani communities. Thus, although once there were no workers from these ethnic groups, now there are; the unwillingness to employ them comes from members of their own community. Unlike the other two ethnic community groups, there is no regular event for the older members served by this project, so a special meeting had to be arranged. The Project also arranged transport and the food which was served at the end of the meeting and which was used to encourage people to participate.

Characteristics of the group

Some people in this group were aged 80 and over, some were younger. There were five males and four females. We have no Barthel scores for this group.

Services currently being used

Unlike the other groups there was a clear recognition in this group of the existence of services provided by the SSD. Three of the nine people were using services provided or purchased by social services on a weekly basis. Only one person in the group did not know about the availability of such services. The services that were being accessed included cleaning, washing and shopping. Two members of the group paid for private help with cooking and shopping.

Asian views on the dimensions of good quality home care services

The group came up with 10 features of a quality home care service; seven of these fell into categories developed in the mainstream study and were all related to what the carers do. Three dimensions had a strong Asian focus.

The Asian dimension

A good quality service is one in which:

- the carer should come later in the day when the Asian shops are open;

- there are permanent staff who know what foods we want, which meat and vegetables;

- food is prepared to suit the individual.

What carers do

A good quality service is one in which:

- carers are honest;

- decorating services are provided;

- a proper bathing service is provided;

- a good massage with cream can be provided;

- carers do their work quickly;

- carers can do cleaning tasks;

- carers can do ironing and washing.

Some methodological issues

The three communities differed both in the way they responded to and participated in the research project. This makes it very clear that working with people from different cultural backgrounds means that the researchers must work flexibly, particularly around the times of events which are an integral part of the communities' own activities. At the same time researchers must try to preserve the integrity of the research method.

There is not only a language problem that needs to be addressed to encourage older people from these communities to express their views, trying to access the views of these groups creates additional difficulties. We received assistance from organisations such as those represented in the BCCCF in Manchester. These organisations act as gatekeepers to different cultural communities in the city and were willing to try out the focus group method for this study. We provided clear explanations of the method and facilitated training. Other relevant issues relate to supporting and encouraging members of these communities to learn the research techniques to enable them to carry out qualitative research of this kind themselves. Additionally, white researchers need to work with members of the community who can make it possible to access the views of older people. There are clearly limits to accessing community groups through these organisations. One route to promoting consultation is to offer training to these groups in the use of these methods and to demonstrate that the information they provide is fed back into service development. It is important that there is some value in the process and the older people in these groups can see the potential outcomes.

The planning of the focus groups in these three different communities took time and did not fit neatly into the timetable for the rest of the research project. This reflects the lack of resources that the people who assisted us have to do this type of work. These groups were actively involved in drafting, planning and implementing the data collection exercise at each stage of the project (they were reimbursed for their services). If involvement and resourcing does not happen, "consultation becomes a meaningless exercise" (Williams and Mussenden, 1992, p 33). In these settings, it is not only that research they have experienced in the past has led to little change in service provision, but also that the service being researched is little known or used by members of these communities. This can generate a distance from the research. A clear limitation of the study of the three groups above is that their members have some connection with formal organisations and may not represent the views of the wider community of which they are a part. The three samples were convenience samples accessed in a particular way and these considerations need to be borne in mind when considering the data.

What we have learnt from this part of the research is that there is overlap in what these older people believe makes a quality home care service with the views of their peers in other communities in the city. However, they also have their own culturally-specific views and can quite clearly make these known if someone takes the time to ask and listen.

5

Accessing older people's views

We used two different ways of obtaining older people's views about the quality of home care services that they would like. In this chapter we describe these methods. We also compare these approaches and identify whether there were differences in the responses obtained by them. We suggest ways to carry out effective group meetings to hear older people's views.

Our two approaches to accessing older people's views were the two-stage focus group and the home-based interview. In both settings we used identical open-ended questions. This type of question provides the opportunity for people to raise their own concerns and come forward with imaginative ideas for the characteristics of a quality service. This way, their needs and views drove the agenda. A recent report from an action research project designed to bring local service providers and older people together to draw up standards and action plans to improve service delivery identified the importance of this approach:

> Open-ended, one-to-one interviews with users proved effective in establishing users' expectations, raising new concerns and stimulating ideas. (National Consumer Council et al, 1999, p 12)

In both settings we also used the technique of paired comparisons, to enable the older people to identify the relative importance, or priority, of the many dimensions of quality they identified.

Advantages and disadvantages of the two methods of accessing older people's views

In Table 1 (page 57) we compare the two methods in terms of:

- the relative cost;

- their use as a source of information;

- their use as a means of setting priorities;

- the length of time they take;

● other benefits and drawbacks.

In the group situation, with a skilled facilitator, considerably more ideas were generated than in the one-to-one interviews in the client's own home. The priority-setting exercise was also considerably harder to do in people's own homes. There were fewer completed sets of paired comparisons in this setting than from the focus groups. This may have been because they were asked to consider other people's ideas about quality or because of the lack of peer support. However, 66% of those interviewed did complete these priority rankings.

The focus groups themselves last a far shorter time on average, even when the provision of food is included, than do interviews. In neither setting have we included travelling time for either clients or the interviewers or staff connected with the focus groups. Another benefit of the focus groups is the pleasure derived from participating experienced by the older people themselves. We began to realise that participating in the focus groups was in and of itself confidence building. It could possibly become a capacity-building process, which may increase their willingness to participate in subsequent implementation and monitoring activities related to the improvement of services.

Difficulties associated with the focus groups are in finding suitable transport and appropriate venues, both of which appear to be extremely thin on the ground. In addition, the significant involvement of a secretary was needed to ensure that participants got to the focus groups. The secretary rang to confirm the availability of participants on the day of the focus group, liaised with the company providing the transport on that day and did other necessary administration.

The benefits for those people who were interviewed at home are that they were not required to leave their own homes, or travel to unknown places in unknown forms of transport. More older people were willing to participate in this way.

Where home interviews occurred, all of the negotiation for these was undertaken by the researchers. The singular disadvantage of the face-to-face interviews was the amount of time the interviewers needed to travel to and from these, and the length of time for carrying out the paired comparisons.

Overall, when these two methods of accessing information are compared in terms of the resource implications, it would appear that the focus group is probably a more efficient way of collecting information. Our data indicate that there is little difference in the information about quality obtained using these two methods.

With finite resources, service providers must make decisions about how they will access older people's views. Our data suggest that using focus groups has advantages and has the additional benefit of building their confidence to participate in further discussions. The focus group also enables the prioritisation process to be carried out more easily than in the homes of older people. However, many older people will not leave their homes to participate in group meetings and it is important to recognise and respect these differences.

The pros and cons of the two methods are summarised in Table 1.

Table 1: Some pros and cons of focus groups and one-to-one interviews as a means of accessing older people's views about the quality of services

Method	Cost	Getting info	Getting priorities	Time (hours)	Other benefits	Other drawbacks
Focus groups	£	✓✓✓	✓✓✓	2-2$\frac{1}{2}$	**	**
Interviews	££	✓✓	✓	$\frac{1}{2}$-3$\frac{1}{2}$	*	*

Note: ✓ = reasonable   ✓✓✓✓ = very good

How to run effective focus groups with older people as key participants

Trying to access older people's views about the quality of home care services has made it clear to us that there are key elements in this process. They are:

- personal contact;
- transport;
- venues;
- personal attention;
- food;
- seating;

- closed communication loops.

All of these must characterise the listening process.

Personal contact

It is important to write to individuals. This needs to be done in a type face and font size that can be read by people with sight impairments. You must assume that a proportion of the clients will not be able to read your letter. Any written communication should be followed up with a telephone call which enables you to establish a personal contact, to ask permission to visit and to explain more clearly what it is that you want their help with. Where older people do not have telephones then a house call is necessary to establish this personal link. This personal contact helps to establish trust and a clearer understanding of why it is important that the older person participates. It also quickly identifies any reasons for non-participation (these can include out-of-date and inaccurate databases held by the local authority, as well as the older person's preference).

Transport

Where home interviews are required the interviewers will need transport and to be able to maintain contact with their office base. Where transport is used to bring older people to locations or group discussions then it is essential that the transport has a tailgate and accommodation suitable for wheelchairs. It is also essential that there is an escort with the transport provided. Finding suitable transport is extremely difficult. We could not get help from local taxi companies or the local authority providers of transport because of their unsuitability and/or their unavailability at the times we needed transport. We used an independent

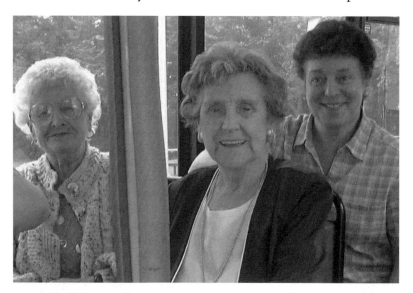

transport provider who was willing to meet our specifications.

It is clearly essential that transport be of the best possible quality. It must be monitored at every stage of the work to ensure that the standard required is maintained.

Venues

Venues for group meetings are as important as transport and are equally difficult to find. They need to be accessible to wheelchairs and have access to kitchen facilities, as well as having suitable toilet facilities. They also need to be flexible. Sometimes it will be necessary, as it was in this project, to sit people round a table and at other times to work with them on a one-to-one basis. The venues need to be located near to people's homes – a maximum journey time of 20 minutes is desirable. Parking close to the entrance to the venue is needed so that older people who are not wheelchair bound, but have difficulty walking, are not disadvantaged. The seating in the venue should be comfortable and there should be somewhere to hang hats and coats. It is also advisable to limit the length of the formal meeting time to an hour-and-a-half, with a short break of 10-15 minutes in the middle.

Personal attention

Personal attention is necessary at the meetings, as it is in the initial contacts, to encourage people to become involved. On the day of the meetings and on the day of the home-based interviews clients were telephoned to ascertain that they would still be available for either the interview or the meeting. At our meetings we used local sixth form students who were assigned to greet and take care of individual participants in the focus groups. This enabled the older people and their partners to build up a relationship and get to know each other. The assistants were responsible for providing cups of tea on the older person's arrival and ensuring that they were given refreshments during the break in the meeting. Additionally, if they needed to go to the toilet they would accompany them if this was necessary. The interaction between the older people and the sixth form students contributed to the pleasantness of the event and minimally added to the cost of running it.

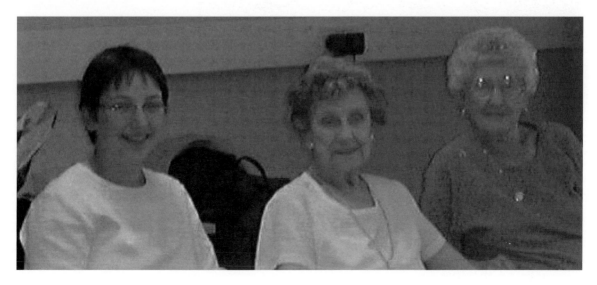

When group members were sitting around a table we used name cards which were clearly printed and computer generated. These should face outwards when people first arrive so that they can see clearly where they are meant to sit. As an icebreaker the cards are turned around and people are then asked to introduce themselves and say how they wish to be addressed at the meeting.

Food

Food is an essential part of running a successful group meeting. Beyond the necessary cup of tea and biscuit at the beginning of the meeting prior to the formal business, it is also a good idea to provide tea with sandwiches and cakes at the end of the meeting. We found a catering service that made delicious bite-sized assorted sandwiches and home-made cakes. These, with strawberries and cream in season, were much enjoyed by all the participants. Tea and coffee was made to their specifications. People were relaxed and enjoyed the simple meal after the hard effort demanded by the focus group. It is advisable to inform the participants that this type of small meal will be provided and to assure them that they will be leaving the venue at a particular time and be returned to their homes by the transport that had been used to get them there. We found that not providing such refreshments seriously reduced the level of participation in the events. We felt that the good humour that eating together engendered was contributory to the willingness of people to continue to be involved in the focus groups.

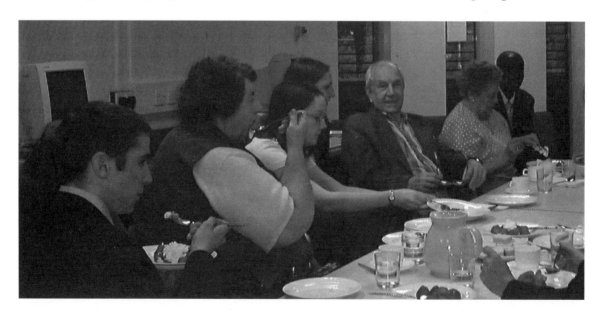

Seating

It is important to ensure that the chairs are comfortable, and that the tables are at the right height to sit around. The positioning of people is also significant in enabling them to participate in what is being discussed. People with hearing difficulties should be seated nearest to the speaker if there is no induction loop available – not everyone has hearing aids. Using a scribe is important because the discussion can be recorded on a flip chart and enables the facilitator to ensure that all of the members of the group participate in the event. It also means that the scribe can regularly repeat, to those who cannot see to read, what is being recorded and check that the written record is a correct one involving all members of the group. We have recorded the group meetings and have not found that there is a significant difference in the information provided from the transcribed tapes and that on the flip chart sheets. The advantage of the latter of course is that it makes the record immediately accessible to all members of the group.

Closed loops

The planning of these group meetings (and indeed the interviews) has to be meticulous with attention being paid to detail. It is important that all of the loops are closed so that a record is kept of the reasons people do not attend meetings or become available for interviews and non-appearances at meetings are followed up and recorded.

Key elements in accessing older people's views using interviews

The use of open-ended questions and the establishment of good rapport will encourage older people to express their views in the interview situation. The same degree of personal attention and negotiation of a suitable time for the interview to take place are important. The provision of clear information about the purpose of the interview and the guarantee of confidentiality will contribute to the development of trust between the interviewer and interviewee. The offer of feedback in the form of the findings from the research will provide the older person with a way of seeing how their contribution fits into the whole picture.

To summarise, we suggest that if listening to what people have to say is to be done successfully, whether it is through an interview in their home or involves them participating in group meetings, attention needs to be given to all the appropriate elements we have described.

6
How to put ideas into practice

As a recent report from the National Consumer Council, Consumer Congress and the Service First Unit in the Cabinet Office has commented, there is now no shortage of guides available on how to consult (Service First, 1998). A clear account of the variety of different ways of consulting with older people is reported in the Better Government for Older People Series (see, for example, Boaz and Hayden, 2000). Many local service providers want to consult their users but doing this effectively is not easy (National Consumer Council, Consumer Congress and Service First Unit, 1999). Going beyond this to involve older people more fully in decisions about the development of the quality of services is more difficult still.

We have discussed the advantages and disadvantages of the methods we have used to access the views of older people. Some of the issues that the older people have raised about the quality of services are ones which could be directly and immediately responded to by SSDs. Other issues go beyond the remit of the SSD within the city in which this research was carried out and deserve consideration on a national level. Some dimensions which the older people identified as important in developing quality services to enable them to live independently in their own home require joined-up solutions. These will involve collaboration and cooperation across service departments, as well as between these departments and commercial organisations such as shops, chemists and communications companies.

One of the aims of this project was to explore the ways in which the views of older people, once they have been accessed, can have an impact on quality specification, so that this service can be subsequently delivered against these specifications. There is no clearly identified system for tracking and using older people's views on the services provided, or for seeing if their views can make a difference to the services delivered.

We began this research with a blank sheet of paper, allowing the older people to define for us what they saw as the quality dimensions of home care services. We did not use a survey – a technique widely used by public service providers and by researchers – because, while it is true that well-designed satisfaction surveys can help to monitor performance and track trend, they are a poor way of uncovering the wider concerns of the individuals who receive home care services. We have argued that the one-to-one interviews and the focus groups are better ways of allowing people to come forward with ideas about the desirable qualities of a home care service.

Accessing the views of service users is now required in the context of Best Value guidance. Consulting people about their views is part of the operation of many local authorities. A series of documents, prepared by the Cabinet Office Service First Group (National Consumer Council et al, 1999), gives advice on how to consult users, and how to involve people so that the delivery of local public services can be improved. Involving older people in specifying the quality of the services they receive at home, to enable them to live there independently means that we must consider three questions:

1. How do we actually hear what older people have to say about the quality of services?

2. How do we input feedback from older people into the setting of quality standards?

3. How do we ensure that older people's contribution (as well as that of the professionals) to the definition of quality standards is actually being delivered?

It is not enough to merely listen to what older people have to say about quality (ie consult with them), it is essential to go beyond this and link the listening to the processes, which inform the delivery and monitoring of home care services. Carter and Beresford (1999) make the point that participation by older people is "not just about different techniques and methods of involving people" (p 11). There are indeed no guarantees that consultation at whatever stage of the development of services will result in the services reflecting the views of users. In trying to ensure that this is the case, it is a prerequisite that all three questions are answered.

How to ensure that the information that older people provide influences practice in setting the standards and is not lost requires finding ways of either fitting this into existing local authority processes or inventing and resourcing new ones.

At the round-table meeting it was concluded that postal surveys, which are now used routinely, contribute some information, but that this method has limited use. This is because some people cannot read the questionnaires, and some are afraid that they will lose services if they complete the questionnaires. Also, the use of postal surveys is a process which does not involve individuals personally. One of the older people in this study pointed out that:

> "In Best Value surveys there are two-and-a-half thousand people's views and you are just one of these – you can't get your view across. This is not the best way of getting individuals' views."

Here are some ideas that could help to ensure that older peoples voices are heard.

> The service providers themselves could be supervised in such a way that the supervisor is able to communicate directly with the older person to ascertain their views.

> The organisers of home care services could ring one service recipient each day to establish that they are getting the services they want and if there are any aspects of it that they think could be improved. This information would then need to be fed into a monitoring system.

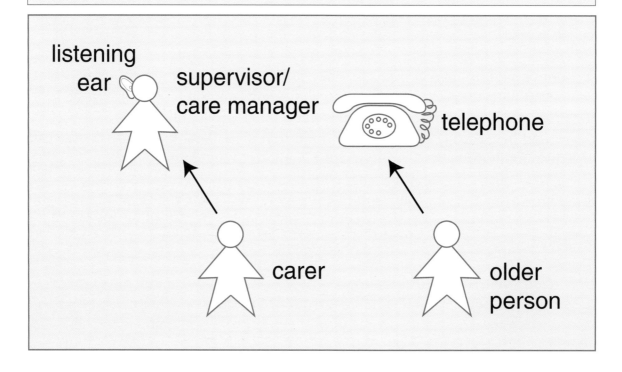

A meeting organised locally two or three times per year would enable managers, social workers and the director of adult services (or the appropriate directorate) to meet with people to learn what is happening in relation to the services being delivered. The independent agency providers could be required, in their service agreements, to come to these events.

The information gleaned from these regular events could be fed into the quality specifications for the service contract.

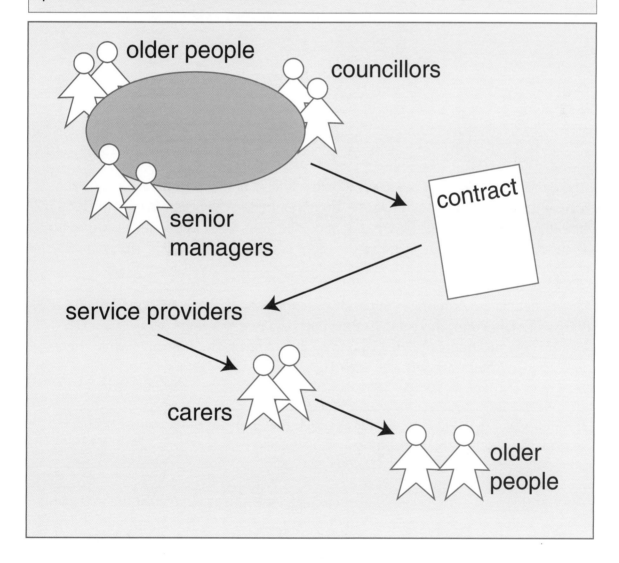

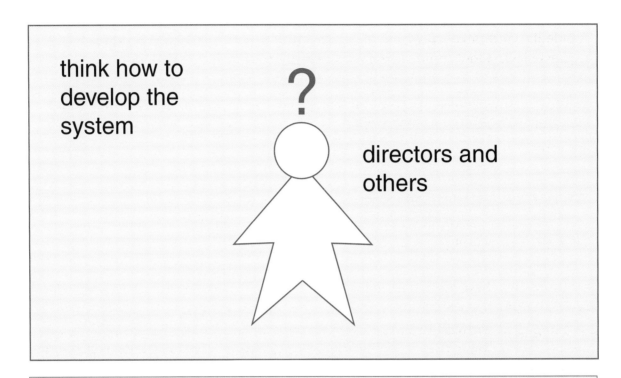

think how to develop the system

?

directors and others

The director for adult services needs to know that all of these events are happening. Thus a system needs to be developed for a) monitoring the occurrence of these activities, and b) using the information provided from them so that it can inform both the setting of quality standards and the monitoring of the delivery of service quality.

Where people are brought together it was suggested that this be done on a patch basis. In Manchester there are 20 such patches. Two meetings per year in each patch could be arranged. Social services could arrange the transport when there is low usage of their transport.

It is important that the time of year at which meetings for older people occur excludes the winter and dark nights.

Courses for carers must include training to teach them to listen to what the user wants.

There should be an annual meeting at the Town Hall to coincide with a tea dance to which older people, councillors, officers and voluntary organisations should come, and the issue of quality of home care services should be the topic for discussion.

Residents' committees based in sheltered accommodation could regularly meet to express views about the quality of service delivered.

Similarly, groups which are based at day centres could meet to express their views, and reflect on the effect of these views on the subsequent quality of services being delivered.

The telephone number of the senior managers for adult services should be at the top of the list of information about services available, which is sent annually to older people receiving home care.

It is clear that there are a number of ways in which older people's ideas can be accessed, but they are all ones in which individuals will need to be personally encouraged to participate and allow their voices to be heard. Senior officers and councillors will have to be literally seen to be listening. Evidence of improvement in the quality of services can be fed back to senior managers through a series of regular meetings. Additionally the more localised information obtained through telephone calls by home care managers and spot checks involving face-to-face interviews by home care supervisors can inform senior managers. There are already groups in place for people in sheltered accommodation and in day care centres. Those who are involved in neither of these can hopefully be encouraged to speak with supervisors or home care managers and be encouraged to come to meetings. A total of 20% of the older people in our study were not available to be spoken to on the telephone; this proportion varied in different parts of the city. Accessing the views of people without access to a telephone requires home visits by home care supervisors or managers.

Accessing older people's views on quality can be integrated into the service specification of quality processes and can, using the same methods, enable the local authority to ascertain if changes to the service specification are being delivered. As one of the senior managers involved in the round-table meeting noted:

> "The presence of regular meetings at which all of the relevant parties – that is, the older people, the service providers, senior managers and councillors – come together, helps enable the senior managers. They can explain when it is not possible and why it is not possible to make the quality changes that people are suggesting."

The problem of users' views having no impact on services will remain unless there is a feedback loop to ensure that change to the services is being delivered. The information gathered from the older people in this study and in subsequent round-table events could be used to feed into the city's documents on standards and quality specifications for the purchase of home care services. Mechanisms need to be established to collect subsequent performance information, review the service delivery procedures and revise the service specifications. It would be sensible and feasible for older people to be involved in all of these activities.

Carter and Beresford (1999) pointed out that if older people do respond to the current government's emphasis in its programmes and policy statements on participation and user involvement, they run the risk of expending much time, energy and resources for little benefit. In the round-table meeting older people generated a number of clear ideas about how their voices could be heard on a regular basis and how their experience of the services delivered could be used to inform a critical appraisal of those services. At the round-table meeting senior managers and elected councillors heard ideas from the older people about possible improvements to the quality of services in their homes. It was noted that some of these could be acted on immediately by senior managers. A case in point was the need to notify the older person if a different carer from the one they were expecting would be coming to their house.

Involving people in the specification of quality standards and the monitoring of their implementation, requires a strategic commitment that would involve all the relevant parts of the SSD and the independent providers of home care services. The mechanisms to enable this to happen in Manchester and elsewhere have been clearly outlined by the older people participating in the round-table meeting.

7 Conclusions and policy implications

There are different types of findings from this study. The first and most important relate to the views of older people about what makes for quality home care services. The second are about ways of continuing to hear what older people say and ensuring their views influence practice. The third findings relate to the infrastructure and the organisation of the services which create the wider understanding of home care services that older people themselves have.

The views of the older people about what makes for quality home care services are very clear. SSDs can immediately address some of these.

Good quality services need to be organised so that:

- people know what their entitlement is;

- service users are informed if there is to be a change in the carer who is coming to their home;

- carers and their reliefs should be consistent so that trust can be built and time saved;

- the timing of the visit or any change in this is notified to the older person;

- the quality of the services is regularly monitored;

- more domestic cleaning is provided;

- the service can be flexible and what is delivered can reflect the individual's wishes, as needs do fluctuate.

The implications of these findings, which were relevant to those both under and over 80 years of age, are that the purchasers need to shift to neighbourhood-based delivery of home care, which is person, rather than task focused.

Thus, the service contract should require that:

● an annual statement of entitlement is sent to older people;

● older people are notified of any change in their carer;

● continuity (ie the same staff providing the service) is a key feature of any personal services delivered.

To monitor the implementation of these dimensions of quality, the proposals from the round-table meetings, which focused on turning ideas into practice, could be tried out. There were essentially two proposals – both involved listening directly to older people. The first suggestion is the provision of regular meetings two or three times per year on a neighbourhood or patch basis, involving providers, senior managers, older people and councillors. This will be successful as long as means are found to feed what they say back into the commissioning, contracting and monitoring systems of the home care services. The second suggestion is the daily monitoring by telephone of one older person per day on a care manager's list. The feedback from this daily event should be reported to a senior designated manager. Following this, a report should be made of any action to be taken, or of reasons why no action will be taken. These suggestions will help the voices of older people to continue to be heard.

Some of the absence of what the older people saw as making for quality services perhaps lies in the underpinning structural arrangements of referral and care management. In a recent report, Sinclair et al (2000) drew attention to the failure of this system to deliver the positive outcomes it was claimed to enable. It clearly does not, as the Kent Community Care Project did, in the 1980s, provide services sensitively and flexibly related to people's wishes and situations. As Sinclair wrote, "It was hard to imagine the needs of older people fell so neatly into half hourly or hourly packages" (p 29). The Kent Project enabled people at local level to purchase flexible patterns of services and such a system could be implemented elsewhere.

Many of the other dimensions identified by older people, as contributing to good quality home care may not be directly accessed by SSDs. This may be because of cash constraints or because of the focus on personal social care. However, local befriending and voluntary groups could be alerted to the importance of visiting and taking people out, as well as undertaking small repairs, odd jobs such as changing light bulbs, or gardening and decorating. The personal social care which is being provided is highly valued and if budget constraints prevent the additional provision of proper cleaning – so often referred to as important – then telling people this is why and seeking alternative delivery systems for it could perhaps help.

Other valued dimensions of quality home care services such as getting out, transport and a universally-available prescription delivery service are not within SSDs' power to deliver. Provision of these will need to involve the health services, transport and police services. Social services can perhaps again act as a voice on behalf of the older people whose needs they address in other ways. No one else does this. Councillors have little access directly to the citizens in their wards, but their knowledge of this more strategic, cross-departmental and inter-agency matter can be informed by SSD managers who listen to older people's views.

Staff who deal with such complex and varied workloads need training, for their benefit, as well as for those for whom they care. The older people in this study clearly value the help they get, but could see how training in all aspects of the job would enhance the quality of the service provided. The training might also bring the status carers deserve. Investment in training has to be long term and the new national standards will set criteria about this. Carers are harder than ever to recruit and retain from a dwindling resource base, when other caring services seek staff from the same source. Considering the development for home care workers of an equivalent to the personal medical services contract currently being piloted in a number of parts of the country, would not only raise their status, but allow them to work as independent contractors. This could assist in the development of something closer to the Kent community care model.

With regards to health, regaining lost senses and physical function remain highly desirable ways of improving the quality of life and individual independence of older people, and therefore of their home care. These are the remit of long-term scientific developments which SSDs can do nothing to expedite, but they loom large in the minds of people over the age of 80. However, ensuring that the prescription collecting, completing and delivery service is a universally available option, should not be beyond the influence of a local authority SSD, especially in the context of the 1999 Health Act (DoH, 1999) and the development of Primary Care Trusts. Time which is now spent by carers collecting prescriptions could be saved and used for other purposes.

The value of sheltered accommodation wardens as a source of monitoring, providing a friendly face each day, and as an optional provider of small services (such as, small repairs and changing lightbulbs), should not be overlooked or undervalued.

Aids and adaptations are valued as adding quality to services. Perhaps integrating the provision of these through the mechanisms of the Primary Care Trusts and the 1999 Health Act, would reduce waiting time for them and ensure they are more readily available.

The vision of the electric buggy in its own lane is one that may seem far-fetched, as might a robot to cut the lawn. However, the latter is now available and it may be that using these as low-level maintenance supports will shortly be financially cost effective. The vision of electric buggies has yet to be realised, but a Department of Health/Department of the Environment, Transport and the Regions joint initiative could turn this into reality at a national level.

The methods for listening

Both our approaches had their pros and cons. No busy SSD has the resources to routinely either conduct home interviews or organise focus groups, notwithstanding the Best Value requirements to consult with service users. However, two issues stand out from this part of our study. First, the accuracy of the database on which any Best Value survey is based has to be questioned, given our experience, especially in the pilot stage of the study. An improvement in data accuracy could be addressed through improved linking of data from charging departments to those of commissioning and assessment. This has serious IT implications for local authorities, but there are cost implications of having the wrong information about older people. Second, electronic improvements to the recouping of charges for services would reduce older people's anxiety, as well as presumably improving the local authority's income stream. As one older person pointed out, direct debit facilities for payment could assist this.

Our face-to-face interviews did not produce dimensions of quality that were not discussed in the focus groups. Thus, it is arguable that interviews are not necessary to obtain accurate and inclusive feedback. Also, the data we have on functional ability (represented by the Barthel scores) shows no significant difference between the groups, although it is possible that those who were interviewed at home, especially those aged over 80, were more likely to be suffering from illness than those who came to focus groups. However, the

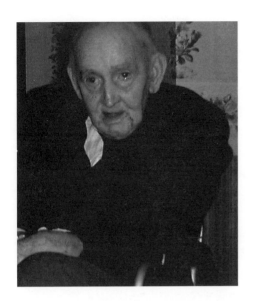

interviews did produce some different prioritising of dimensions. Providing the opportunity for this group to contribute has two gains: the views of more people could be listened to and the views of people who rarely contribute would be heard. It is true that a small number of very disabled people with sensory difficulties and physical disabilities came to the focus groups and these events can be accessible to more people if suitable venues and transport are provided. However, the focus groups have two other advantages: they are clearly sociable occasions for older people and they seem to act as a capacity-building event in their own right for those who participated. Either approach will have its problems: we had a high rate of refusal, and, unfortunately, death contributed to our low participation rate.

However, research should continue to focus on listening to older people in order to improve the dimensions of the quality of home care services. There is scope for implementing changes in the processes that make up home care services, the systems that deliver them and those other dimensions of daily life that go to make up quality services as defined by the older people to whom we have been privileged to listen.

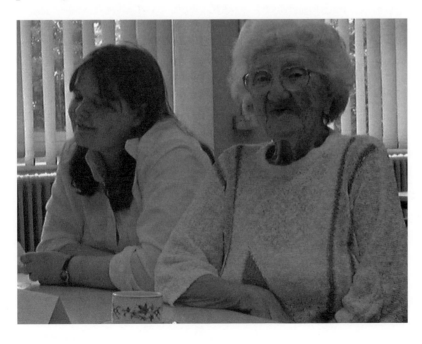

References

Boaz, A. and Hayden, C. (2000) *Listening to local older people*, Coventry: University of Warwick.

Carter, T. and Beresford, P. (1999) *Models of involvement for older people*, York: Joseph Rowntree Foundation.

Challis, D. and Davies, B. (1986) *Case management in community care*, Aldershot: Gower.

CIPFA (Chartered Institute of Public Finance and Accountancy) (1998) *Personal social services statistics: 1996-97 Actuals*, London: CIPFA.

CIPFA (1999) *Personal social services statistics: 1997-98 Actuals*, London: CIPFA.

DoH (Department of Health) (1989) *Caring for people: Community care in the next decade and beyond*, London: HMSO.

DoH (1999) *Health Act*, London: HMSO.

Edelbalk, P.G., Samuelsson, G. and Ingvad, B. (1995) 'How elderly people rank-order the quality characteristics of home services', *Ageing and Society*, vol 15 no 1, pp 83-103.

Godfrey, M., Randall, T., Long, A. and Grant, M. (2000) *Review of effectiveness and outcomes: Home care*, Exeter: University of Exeter.

Gordon, J., Powell, C. and Rockwood, K. (1999) 'Goal attainment scaling as a measure of clinically important change in nursing-home patients', *Age and Ageing*, vol 28, no 3, pp 275-81.

Hayden, C. and Boaz, A. (2000) *The Better Government for Older People Programme evaluation report: Making a difference*, Coventry: Local Government Centre/Warwick University.

Henwood, M., Lewis, H. and Waddington, E. (1998) *Listening to users of domiciliary care services*, Leeds: Nuffield Institute for Health Community Care Division.

Initiatives in Care (2000) *National standards for regulating organisations providing domiciliary care*, Draft 8, London: DoH.

Jarman, B. (1983) 'Identification of underprivileged areas', *British Medical Journal*, no 286, pp 1705-9.

National Consumer Council, Consumer Congress and Service First Unit (1999) *Involving users: Improving the delivery of local public services*, London: Cabinet Office.

OPCS (Office for Population, Censuses and Surveys) (1996) *Living in Britain 1994: General household survey*, London: HMSO.

Public Health Directorate (1996) *Manchester public health annual report*, Manchester: Manchester Health Authority.

Qureshi, H., Patmore, C., Nicholas, E. and Bamford, C. (1999) *Overview: Outcomes of social care for older people and carers*, Outcomes in Community Care Practice No 5, York: Social Policy Research Unit, University of York.

Radar and Arthritis Care (1991) *A right to a clean home*, London: Radar/Arthritis Care.

Service First (1998) *An introductory guide: How to consult your users*, London: Cabinet Office.

Sinclair, I., Gibbs, I. and Hicks, L. (2000) *The management and effectiveness of the home care services*, York: Social Work Research and Development Unit, University of York.

SSI (Social Services Inspectorate) (1987) *From home help to home care: An analysis of policy, resources and service management*, London: SSI/Department of Health and Social Security.

Williams, E. and Mussenden, B. (1992) 'Community care and consultation with black and minority ethnic communities', *Critical Public Health*, vol 3, no 4, pp 31-5.

Woodruff, L. and Applebaum, R. (1996) 'Assuring the quality of in-home supportive services: a consumer perspective', *Journal of Ageing Studies*, vol 10, no 2, pp 137-69.

Appendix

The original sample obtained in November 1999 came from a social services database which contained details of people for whom home care services were being purchased by Manchester City Council. The database was organised into Primary Care Group areas (address/ward) and by age groups (by date of birth). A random 10% sample of names was selected using random numbers generated by using a calculator. Once the names had been selected for the sample they were forwarded to Manchester SSD to check that the individual selected was still receiving home care services.

In the pilot phase of the project it became apparent that the database from which the sample had been selected in December 1999 included a large number of people who had died and often gave inaccurate contact information. During the pilot we also identified the fact that many older people would not come to the focus groups. These groups had been designed to be the primary source of data for the study. At this stage it was decided to offer home-based interviews to older people who would not come to the planned meetings. We discussed with members of the Steering Group the problems we had had with the population database. However, 1,000 more older people had been added to the database in the six months since we had received it and drawn our original sample, and the problems about locating older people were also resolved. The problems appeared to derive from the existence of two separate databases which were in operation in different parts of the SSD. It was agreed that we would use the updated version of the database from which to draw the sample for the rest of the study. This new population database obtained in January 2000 provided us with fewer, but still a considerable number of contact problems. We have corrected the database in the course of the study (for example, reducing the number of records indicating no telephone in home from 50% to 20%). However a large number of those in the sample were still not able to participate in the study or refused to. Table A1 shows the difficulties of finding appropriate people to participate in the study.

Table A1: Attrition in sample size

Total number of participants from original sampling frame	**292**
Non-contactable/deceased/ill/inappropriate selection	**74**
Total possible participants	**218**

Table A2 shows that the refusal rate was relatively high, however, and Figure A1 shows that the participation rate was just under 50%.

Table A2: Refusal

Number of participants that attended focus groups	39
Number of participants that attended interviews	64
Number of participants that refused	114

Focus groups and interviews

A total of 12 first-stage focus groups and 10 second-stage focus groups were held. It was possible to consolidate groups at stage two when the paired comparisons were being made. A total of 39 people were involved in these focus groups, and 64 people in the interviews. Figure A1 shows the proportions and reflects the non-participant level of 53% (114 people).

Figure A1: Participants that attended a focus group, had an interview or refused

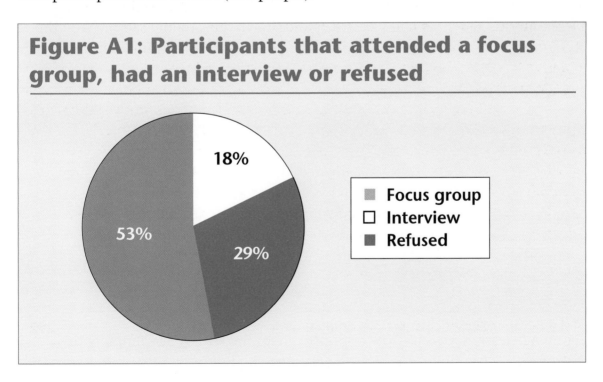

Functional assessment

We had hoped to be able to compare our population in the study with that in other studies in terms of their functional ability. We also thought that it would aid us in determining if the population that came to the focus groups and those who wanted to be interviewed in their own homes differed.

We chose, after much discussion, to use the Barthel questionnaire since this appeared to provide not only a well established but also a relatively quick means of obtaining an assessment of the capabilities of the participants in the study. It was not possible for these to be completed by the carers or the participants' families. Involving the carers would have been extremely complex as well as violating the commitment to confidentiality which has been maintained. Also, many people lived by themselves. A decision was made to ask the participants to complete the questionnaires themselves. However, this has resulted in a very small number of questionnaires being returned: 11 from those involved in the focus groups and 43 from those involved in the interviews.

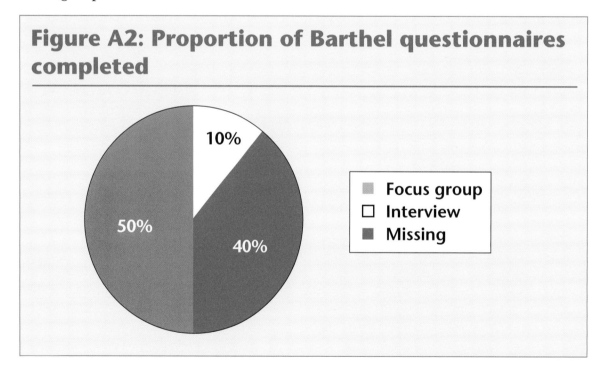

Figure A2: Proportion of Barthel questionnaires completed

Figure A2 clearly shows the low response rate to the request to complete this instrument. The questionnaire itself appears to be not only difficult to use in this context, but also insensitive to the sensory disabilities we observed which were as disabling as any of the physical disabilities it identified. Others have identified the limitations of the measure (see Gordon et al, 1999). As a proxy for measurement of functional ability we recorded the information we have about the number of hours of service provided by the home care agencies involved. Neither this nor the Barthel data indicate any significant differences in the population who came to the focus groups and those who were interviewed at home.

Prioritising the features of quality

The participants ranked the statements of quality that had been identified in the first set of focus groups as desirable in home care services. The technique of paired comparisons was used to do this. The rank given by each older person for each statement was then totalled. This gave us the ranking overall for each element of quality.

The statements made by the older people about what constitutes quality in home care services were then categorised and we have called these categories the dimensions of quality. The ranking process enabled us to determine which dimensions were of highest priority for them.